The Respiratory System at a Glance

The Respiratory System at a Glance

Jeremy P.T. Ward

PhD
Professor of Respiratory Cell Physiology
Division of Asthma, Allergy and Lung Biology
King's College London School of Medicine
London, UK

Jane Ward

MBChB, PhD
Senior Lecturer
Division of Physiology
King's College London
London, UK

Richard M. Leach

MD, FRCP
Consultant Physician and Honorary Senior Lecturer
Guy's and St Thomas' Hospital Trust and
King's College London School of Medicine
St Thomas' Hospital
London, UK

Charles M. Wiener

MD
Professor of Medicine and Physiology
Department of Medicine
Johns Hopkins School of Medicine
Baltimore MD, USA

Second edition

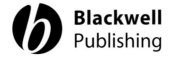
Blackwell
Publishing

© 2006 J.P.T. Ward, J. Ward, R.M. Leach, C.M. Weiner
Published by Blackwell Publishing Ltd
Blackwell Publishing, Inc., 350 Main Street, Malden, Massachusetts 02148-5020, USA
Blackwell Publishing Ltd, 9600 Garsington Road, Oxford OX4 2DQ, UK
Blackwell Publishing Asia Pty Ltd, 550 Swanston Street, Carlton, Victoria 3053, Australia

First published 2002
Second edition 2006

2   2007

Library of Congress Cataloging-in-Publication Data

The respiratory system at a glance / Jeremy P.T. Ward . . . [et al.]. – 2nd ed.
   p. ; cm. -- (At a glance series)
Includes index.
ISBN 978-1-4051-3448-4 (alk. paper)
1. Respiratory organs–Diseases.   I. Ward, Jeremy P. T.   II. Series: At a glance series (Oxford, England)
[DNLM: 1. Respiratory Physiology.   2. Respiratory System–physiopathology.   3. Respiratory Tract Diseases.   WF 102 R437 2006]
RC731.R493   2006
616.2–dc22

                                                                        2006002001

ISBN 978-1-4051-3448-4

A catalogue record for this title is available from the British Library

Set in 9 on 11.5pt Times New Roman PS by SNP Best-set Typesetter Ltd., Hong Kong
Printed and bound in Singapore by Markono Print Media Pte Ltd

Commissioning Editor: Martin Sugden
Development Editor: Geraldine Jeffers
Production Controller: Kate Charman

For further information on Blackwell Publishing, visit our website:
http://www.blackwellpublishing.com

The publisher's policy is to use permanent paper from mills that operate a sustainable forestry policy, and which has been manufactured from pulp processed using acid-free and elementary chlorine-free practices. Furthermore, the publisher ensures that the text paper and cover board used have met acceptable environmental accreditation standards.

Contents

Preface to second edition

The medical curriculum has become increasingly vertically integrated, with a much greater use of clinical examples and cases to help in the understanding of the relevance of the underlying basic science, and conversely use of basic science concepts to help in the understanding of the pathophysiology and treatment of disease. *The Respiratory System at a Glance* has been written to take account of this trend, and to integrate core aspects of basic science, pathophysiology and treatment into a single, easy to use revision aid. As such, it should be useful to medical students throughout their training, and also to other healthcare professions, including nursing.

As with other volumes in the *At a Glance* series, it is based around a two-page spread for each main topic, with figures and text complementing each other to give an overview of a topic at a glance. Case studies based on some of the most commonly encountered conditions are also provided, and can be used for both basic science and clinical study. Although primarily designed for revision, the book covers all the core elements of the respiratory system and its major diseases, and as such could be used as a main text in the first couple of years of the course. It is advised, however, that additional reference to more detailed textbooks will aid deeper and wider understanding of the subject. This is particu-larly the case for the pathophysiological chapters, as a book of this length cannot hope to provide a complete guide to clinical practice.

This second edition includes some additional topics requested by our readers (such as exercise, history taking and examination, and an expanded section on pneumonia), and most of the other chapters have been completely revised and updated. The figures have also been revised to make them easier to comprehend, with additional and/or better X-rays/CT scans. Hopefully, we have also corrected the more ridiculous errors found in the last edition. We have been greatly assisted in this by our many colleagues and students who have kindly advised us and commented on the contents, but any remaining errors and omissions are entirely our responsibility. We would also like to thank all the staff at Blackwell Publishing, in particular Geraldine Jeffers; without her excellent advice and enthusiasm we would not have been able to produce this second edition on time.

Jeremy Ward
Jane Ward
Richard Leach
Charles Wiener

Units and symbols

Units

The medical profession and scientific community generally use SI (Système International) units.

Pressure conversion: SI unit of pressure: 1 pascal $(Pa) = 1\,N \cdot m^{-2}$. As this is small, in medicine the kPa $(=10^3\,Pa)$ is more commonly used. Note that millimetres of mercury (mmHg) are still the most common unit for expressing arterial and venous blood pressures, and low pressures — e.g. central venous pressure and intrapleural pressure — are sometimes expressed as centimetres of H_2O (cmH_2O). Blood gas partial pressures are reported by some laboratories in kPa and by some in mmHg, so you need to be familiar with both systems.

$1\,kPa = 7.5\,mmHg = 10.2\,cmH_2O$
$1\,mmHg = 1\,torr = 0.133\,kPa = 1.36\,cmH_2O$
$1\,cmH_2O = 0.098\,kPa = 0.74\,mmHg$
1 standard atmosphere $(\approx 1\ bar) = 101.3\,kPa = 760\,mmHg = 1033\,cmH_2O$

Contents are still commonly expressed per 100 mL (dL^{-1}), and these need to be multiplied by 10 to give the more standard SI unit per litre. Contents are also increasingly being expressed as $mmol \cdot L^{-1}$.

For haemoglobin: $1\,g \cdot dL^{-1} = 10\,g \cdot L^{-1} = 0.062\,mmol \cdot L^{-1}$
For ideal gases (including oxygen and nitrogen): 1 mmol = 22.4 mL standard temperature and pressure dry (STPD; see Chapter 4)
For non-ideal gases, such as nitrous oxide and carbon dioxide: 1 mmol = 22.25 mL STPD

Symbols

Symbols used in respiratory and cardiovascular physiology are given in Fig. 4 (Chapter 4)

Typical inspired, alveolar and blood gas values in healthy young adults are shown in the table below. Ranges are given for arterial blood gas values. Mean arterial P_{O_2} falls with age, and by 60 years is about 11 kPa/82 mmHg. Typical values for lung volumes and other lung function tests are given in the appropriate chapters. Ranges for many values are affected by age, sex and height, as well as by the method of measurement, and hence it is necessary to refer to appropriate nomograms.

Inspired P_{O_2} (dry, sea level)	21 kPa	159 mmHg
Alveolar P_{O_2}	13.3 kPa	100 mmHg
Arterial P_{O_2}	12.5 (11.2–13.9) kPa	94 (84–104) mmHg
A–a P_{O_2} gradient	<2 kPa	<15 mmHg (greater in elderly)
Oxygen saturation	>97%	
Oxygen content	$20\,mL \cdot dL^{-1}$	
Inspired P_{CO_2}	0.03 kPa	0.2 mmHg
Alveolar P_{CO_2}	5.3 (4.7–6.1) kPa	40 (35–45) mmHg
Arterial P_{CO_2}	5.3 (4.7–6.1) kPa	40 (35–45) mmHg
Arterial CO_2 content	$48\,mL \cdot dL^{-1}$	
Arterial $[H^+]$/pH	36–$44\,nmol \cdot L^{-1}$/ 7.44–7.36	
Resting mixed venous P_{O_2}	5.3 kPa	40 mmHg
Resting mixed venous O_2 content	$15\,mL \cdot dL^{-1}$	
Resting oxygen saturation	75%	
Resting mixed venous P_{CO_2}	6.1 kPa	46 mmHg
Resting mixed venous CO_2 content	$52\,mL \cdot dL^{-1}$	
Arterial $[HCO_3^-]$	24 (21–27) mM	

List of abbreviations

A–a gradient	(A–a Po_2) gradient, the difference between ideal alveolar and arterial Po_2
AAT	α_1-antitrypsin
AHI	apnoea plus hypopnoea index
AIDS	acquired immune deficiency syndrome
AIP	acute interstitial pneumonia/pneumonitis (Hamman–Rich syndrome)
ALI	acute lung injury
ANA	anti-nuclear antibody
ANCA	anti-neutrophil cytoplasmic antibody
AP	anterior–posterior
ARDS	acute (formerly adult) respiratory distress syndrome
ATPS	ambient temperature and pressure saturated
ATS	American Thoracic Society (guidelines)
BAL	bronchoalveolar lavage
BALT	bronchus-associated lymphoid tissue
BCG	bacille Calmette–Guérin
BiPAP	bilevel positive airway pressure, biphasic positive airway pressure
BP	blood pressure
BTPS	body temperature and pressure saturated
BTS	British Thoracic Society (guidelines)
CA	carbonic anhydrase
cAMP	cyclic adenosine monophosphate
CAP	community-acquired pneumonia
CCF	congestive cardiac failure
CF	cystic fibrosis
CFA	cryptogenic fibrosing alveolitis
CFTR	cystic fibrosis transmembrane conductance regulator
C_L	lung compliance $= \Delta V/\Delta P$, where P = alveolar–intrapleural pressure
CMV	controlled mechanical ventilation
CMV	cytomegalovirus
CNS	central nervous system
COAD	chronic obstructive airway disease (synonymous with COPD, COLD)
COLD	chronic obstructive lung disease (synonymous with COAD, COPD)
COPD	chronic obstructive pulmonary disease (synonymous with COAD, COLD)
COX	cyclooxygenase
CPAP	continuous positive airway pressure
CREST	calcinosis, Raynaud's phenomenon, esophageal involvement, sclerodactyly, and telangiectasi
CSA	central sleep apnoea
CSF	cerebrospinal fluid
CT	computed tomography
CTPA	computed tomography pulmonary angiogram
CWP	coal worker's pneumoconiosis
CXR	chest X-ray
DIP	desquamative interstitial pneumonia
$D_L$co	diffusing capacity of the lungs for carbon monoxide
D_Lg	diffusing capacity of the lungs for gas
D_Lo$_2$	diffusing capacity of the lungs for oxygen
DRG	dorsal respiratory group
DVT	deep veous thrombosis
EBV	Epstein–Barr virus
ECG	electrocardiogram
ECMO	extracorporeal membrane oxygenation
ECP	eosinophil cationic protein
EEG	electroencephalogram
EGF	epidermal growth factor
ELISA	enzyme-linked immunoassay
EMG	electromyogram
EOG	electrooculogram
ERV	expiratory reserve volume
ESR	erythrocyte sedimentation rate
FDG	fluorodeoxyglucose
FDG PET	fluorodeoxyglucose positron emission tomography
FEF$_{25-75}$	mean forced expiratory flow over middle 50% of forced vital capacity
FER	forced expiratory ratio
FEV$_1$	forced expiratory volume in 1 second
FEV$_1$/FVC	FEV$_1$ expressed as a fraction, or more usually a percentage of FVC (= FER)
FGF	fibroblast growth factor
FRC	functional residual capacity
FVC	forced vital capacity
GBM	glomerular basement membrane
GM-CSF	granulocyte macrophage colony-stimulating factor
GU	genitourinary
HAART	highly active antiretroviral therapy
HAP	hospital acquired pneumonia
HCAP	healthcare-associated pneumonia
HIV	human immunodeficiency virus
HR	heart rate
HRCT	high-resolution computed tomography
ICU	intensive care unit
IFN-γ	interferon-γ
Ig	immunoglobulin, e.g. IgA, IgE, IgG, IgM
IL	interleukin, e.g. IL-10
ILD	interstitial lung disease
INPV	intermittent negative pressure ventilation
IPF	idiopathic pulmonary fibrosis (synonymous with CFA)
IPPV	intermittent positive pressure breathing
IRV	inspiratory reserve volume
IVC	inferior vena cava
JVP	jugular venous pressure
Kco	$D_L$co divided by alveolar volume or Krough coefficient
KS	Kaposi's sarcoma
LA	left atrium, left atrial
LDH	lactate dehydrogenase
LG	lymphomatoid granulomatosis
LIP	lymphocytic interstitial pneumonia
LMWH	low molecular weight heparin
LT	leukotriene, e.g. LTC$_4$
LV	left ventricle, left ventricular
MBP	major basic protein
MDR	multidrug resistant
MI	myocardial infarction
MIE	meconium ileus equivalent
MMV	mandatory minute ventilation
MOF	multiorgan failure
MRSA	methicillin resistant *Staphylococcus aureus*
MVV	maximal voluntary ventilation
NANC	non-adrenergic, non-cholinergic (nerves)
NHL	non-Hodgkin's lymphoma
NIPPV	non-invasive positive pressure ventilation
NRDS	neonatal respiratory distress syndrome
NREM	non-rapid eye movement

NSAID non-steroidal anti-inflammatory drug
NSC non-small cell
NSIP non-specific interstitial pneumonia
OSA obstructive sleep apnoea
P_{50} partial pressure at which haemoglobin is 50% saturated with O_2
P_A alveolar pressure
PA posterior–anterior
PA pulmonary arterial
$P_A CO$ partial pressure of carbon monoxide in the alveoli
$P_a CO_2$ arterial partial pressure of carbon dioxide
$P_A CO_2$ alveolar partial pressure of CO_2
PAF platelet-activating factor
$P_a O_2$ partial pressure of oxygen in the arterial blood
PAV pulmonary arterial vasculopathy (formerly primary pulmonary hypertension)
PCP *Pneumocystis carinii* pneumonia
$PD_{20}FEV_1$ provocative dose (e.g. of histamine or methacholine) that induces a 20% fall in FEV_1
PDGF platelet-derived growth factor
PE pulmonary embolus, pulmonary embolism
PEEP positive end-expiratory pressure
PEFR peak expiratory flow rate
PET positron emission tomography
Pg prostaglandin, e.g. PgD_2
PH pulmonary hypertension
pHa arterial pH
pK_A log of dissociation constant K_A
PMF progressive massive fibrosis
PMI point of maximal impulse (also known as Apex beat)
PPD purified protein derivative
PPHN persistent pulmonary hypertension of the newborn
PSP primary spontaneous pneumothorax
R respiratory gas exchange ratio
RAD right axis deviation (electrocardiography)
RANTES regulated on activation normal T cell expressed and secreted
RAW airway resistance (mouth–alveolar pressure/airflow)
RBBB right bundle branch block
RBC red blood cell
REM rapid eye movement
RV residual volume
RV right ventricle
RVD restrictive ventilatory defect
$S_a O_2$ oxygen saturation of arterial blood (%)
SC small cell
SCUBA self-contained underwater breathing apparatus
SIADH syndrome of inappropriate secretion of anti-diuretic hormone
SIMV synchronized intermittent mandatory ventilation
SLE systemic lupus erythematosus
SO_2 oxygen saturation (oxygen content/oxygen capacity)
SP surfactant protein, e.g. SP-A
STPD standard temperature and pressure dry
SVC superior vena cava
TB tuberculosis
TGFβ transforming growth factor β
TLC total lung capacity
$T_L CO$ carbon monoxide transfer factor (alternative name for $D_L CO$)
UFH unfractionated heparin
UIP usual interstitial pneumonia
VAP ventilator-associated pneumonia
V_A/Q ventilation–perfusion ratio (alveolar ventilation/blood flow in a lung region)
VC vital capacity
VEGF vascular endothelial growth factor
VIP vasoactive intestinal peptide
$\dot{V}O_2$ **max** maximum oxygen consumption
VRG ventral respiratory groups
V_T tidal volume
WBC white blood cell
WCC white cell count
WG Wegener's granulomatosis

Structure of the respiratory system: lungs, airways and dead space

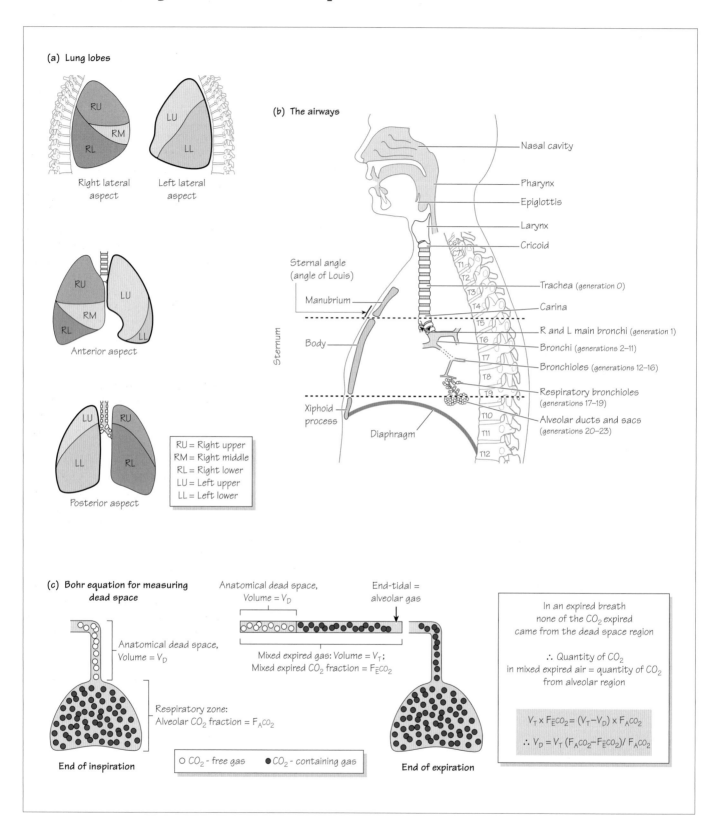

(a) Lung lobes

Right lateral aspect — Left lateral aspect

Anterior aspect

Posterior aspect

RU = Right upper
RM = Right middle
RL = Right lower
LU = Left upper
LL = Left lower

(b) The airways

Nasal cavity
Pharynx
Epiglottis
Larynx
Cricoid
Sternal angle (angle of Louis)
Manubrium
Trachea (generation 0)
Carina
Body
R and L main bronchi (generation 1)
Bronchi (generations 2–11)
Bronchioles (generations 12–16)
Respiratory bronchioles (generations 17–19)
Xiphoid process
Alveolar ducts and sacs (generations 20–23)
Diaphragm
Sternum

(c) Bohr equation for measuring dead space

Anatomical dead space, Volume = V_D

End-tidal = alveolar gas

Anatomical dead space, Volume = V_D

Mixed expired gas: Volume = V_T;
Mixed expired CO_2 fraction = $F_{\bar{E}}CO_2$

Respiratory zone:
Alveolar CO_2 fraction = F_ACO_2

End of inspiration

○ CO_2 - free gas ● CO_2 - containing gas

End of expiration

In an expired breath
none of the CO_2 expired
came from the dead space region

∴ Quantity of CO_2
in mixed expired air = quantity of CO_2
from alveolar region

$$V_T \times F_{\bar{E}}CO_2 = (V_T - V_D) \times F_ACO_2$$

$$\therefore V_D = V_T (F_ACO_2 - F_{\bar{E}}CO_2)/ F_ACO_2$$

Lungs

The respiratory system consists of a pair of **lungs** within the **thoracic cage** (Chapter 2). Its main function is gas exchange, but other roles include speech, filtration of microthrombi arriving from systemic veins and metabolic activities such as conversion of angiotensin I to angiotensin II and removal or deactivation of serotonin, bradykinin, norepinephrine, acetylcholine and drugs such as propranolol and chlorpromazine. The **right lung** is divided by **transverse and oblique fissures** into three lobes: upper, middle and lower. The **left lung** has an **oblique fissure** and two lobes (Fig. 1a). Vessels, nerves and lymphatics enter the lungs on their medial surfaces at the lung root or **hilum**. Each lobe is divided into a number of wedge-shaped **bronchopulmonary segments** with their apices at the hilum and bases at the lung surface. Each bronchopulmonary segment is supplied by its own segmental bronchus, artery and vein and can be removed surgically with little bleeding or air leakage from the remaining lung.

The **pulmonary nerve plexus** lies behind each hilum, receiving fibres from both **vagi** and the second to fourth thoracic **ganglia** of the **sympathetic trunk**. Each vagus contains sensory afferents from lungs and airways and parasympathetic bronchoconstrictor and secretomotor efferents. Sympathetic fibres are bronchodilator but relatively sparse.

Each lung is lined by a thin membrane, the **visceral pleura**, which is continuous with the **parietal pleura**, lining the chest wall, diaphragm, pericardium and mediastinum. The space between the parietal and visceral layers is tiny in health and lubricated with pleural fluid. The right and left pleural cavities are separate and each extends as the **costodiaphragmatic recess** below the lungs even during full inspiration. The parietal pleura is segmentally innervated by **intercostal nerves** and by the **phrenic nerve**, and so pain from pleural inflammation (**pleurisy**) is often referred to the chest wall or shoulder tip. The visceral pleura lacks sensory innervation.

Lymph channels are absent in alveolar walls, but accompany small blood vessels conveying lymph towards the hilar **bronchopulmonary nodes** and from there to **tracheobronchial nodes** at the tracheal bifurcation. Some lymph from the lower lobe drains to the **posterior mediastinal nodes**.

The **upper respiratory tract** consists of the nose, pharynx and larynx. The **lower respiratory tract** (Fig. 1b) starts with the trachea at the lower border of the **cricoid cartilage**, level with the sixth cervical vertebra (C6). It bifurcates into **right and left main bronchi** at the level of the **sternal angle** and T4/5 (lower when upright and in inspiration). The right main bronchus is wider, shorter and more vertical than the left, so inhaled foreign bodies enter it more easily.

Airways

The airways divide repeatedly, with each successive **generation** approximately doubling in number. The **trachea** and **main bronchi** have U-shaped cartilage linked posteriorly by smooth muscle. Lobar bronchi supply the three right and two left lung lobes and divide to give **segmental bronchi** (generations 3 and 4). The total cross-sectional area of each generation is minimum here, after which it rises rapidly, as increased numbers more than make up for their reduced size. Generations 5–11 are small bronchi, the smallest being 1 mm in diameter. The lobar, segmental and small bronchi are supported by irregular plates of cartilage, with bronchial smooth muscle forming helical bands. **Bronchioles** start at about generation 12 and from this point on cartilage is absent. These airways are embedded in lung tissue, which holds them open like tent guy ropes. The **terminal bronchioles** (generation 16) lead to **respiratory bronchioles**, the first generation to have alveoli (Chapter 5) in their walls. These lead to **alveolar ducts** and **alveolar sacs** (generation 23), whose walls are entirely composed of **alveoli**.

The bronchi and airways down to the terminal bronchioles receive nutrition from the **bronchial arteries** arising from the descending aorta. The respiratory bronchioles, alveolar ducts and sacs are supplied by the **pulmonary circulation** (Chapter 13).

The airways from trachea to respiratory bronchioles are lined with **ciliated columnar epithelial cells**. **Goblet cells** and **submucosal glands** secrete **mucus**. Synchronous beating of cilia moves the mucus and associated debris to the mouth (**mucociliary clearance**) (Chapter 18). Epithelial cells forming the walls of alveoli and alveolar ducts are unciliated, and largely very thin **type I alveolar pneumocytes** (alveolar cells; *squamous epithelium*). These form the gas exchange surface with the capillary endothelium (**alveolar-capillary membrane**). A few **type II pneumocytes** secrete **surfactant** which reduces surface tension and prevents alveolar collapse (Chapters 6 & 18).

Dead space

The upper respiratory tract and airways as far as the terminal bronchioles do not take part in gas exchange. These **conducting airways** form the **anatomical dead space** (V_D), whose volume is normally about 150 mL. These airways have an air-conditioning function, warming, filtering and humidifying inspired air.

Alveoli that have lost their blood supply—for example because of a **pulmonary embolus**—no longer take part in gas exchange and form **alveolar dead space**. The sum of the anatomical and alveolar dead space is known as the **physiological dead space**, ventilation of which is wasted in terms of gas exchange. In health, all alveoli take part in gas exchange, so physiological dead space equals anatomical dead space.

The volume of a breath or **tidal volume** (V_T), is about 500 mL at rest. Resting **respiratory frequency** (f) is about 15 breaths/min, so the volume entering the lungs each minute, the **minute ventilation** ($\dot{V}$) is about 7500 mL/min (=500 × 15) at rest. **Alveolar ventilation** ($\dot{V}_A$) is the volume taking part in gas exchange each minute. At rest, dead space volume = 150 mL and alveolar ventilation is 5250 mL/min (=(500–150) × 15).

The **Bohr method** for measuring anatomical dead space is based on the principle that the degree to which dead space gas (0% CO_2) dilutes alveolar gas (about 5% CO_2) to give mixed expired gas (about 3.5%) depends on its volume (Fig. 1c). **Alveolar gas** can be sampled at the end of the breath as **end-tidal gas**. The Bohr equation can be modified to measure physiological dead space by using arterial $P\text{CO}_2$ to estimate the CO_2 in the gas-exchanging or **ideal alveoli**.

2 The thoracic cage and respiratory muscles

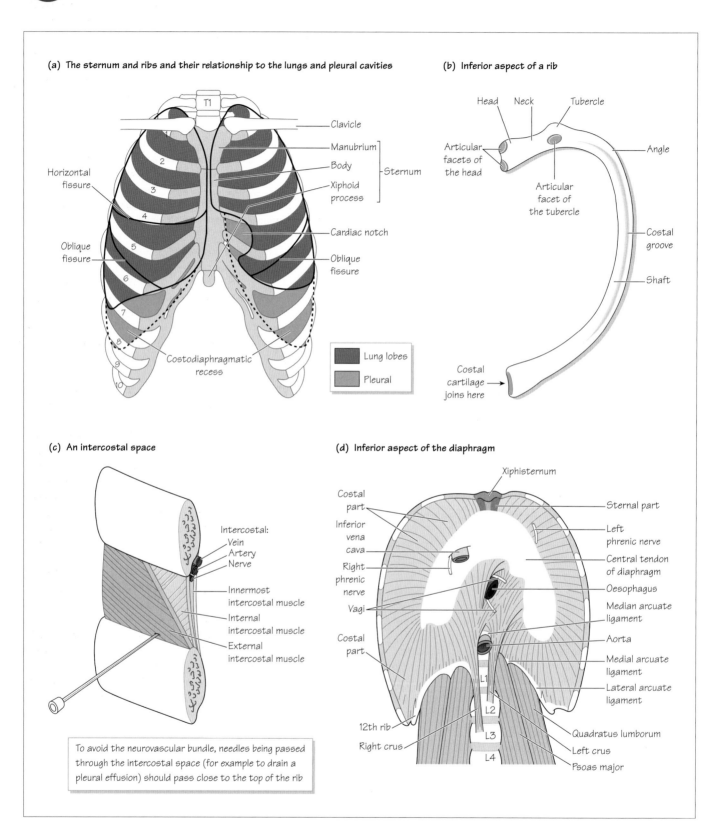

(a) The sternum and ribs and their relationship to the lungs and pleural cavities

T1

Clavicle

Manubrium

Body

Xiphoid process

⎤ Sternum

Horizontal fissure

Oblique fissure

Cardiac notch

Oblique fissure

Costodiaphragmatic recess

Lung lobes

Pleural

(b) Inferior aspect of a rib

Head   Neck   Tubercle

Articular facets of the head

Articular facet of the tubercle

Angle

Costal groove

Shaft

Costal cartilage joins here

(c) An intercostal space

Intercostal:
Vein
Artery
Nerve

Innermost intercostal muscle

Internal intercostal muscle

External intercostal muscle

To avoid the neurovascular bundle, needles being passed through the intercostal space (for example to drain a pleural effusion) should pass close to the top of the rib

(d) Inferior aspect of the diaphragm

Xiphisternum

Costal part

Inferior vena cava

Right phrenic nerve

Vagi

Costal part

12th rib

Right crus

L1

L2

L3

L4

Sternal part

Left phrenic nerve

Central tendon of diaphragm

Oesophagus

Median arcuate ligament

Aorta

Medial arcuate ligament

Lateral arcuate ligament

Quadratus lumborum

Left crus

Psoas major

Thoracic cage

The **thoracic cage** is composed of the **sternum, ribs, intercostal spaces** and **thoracic vertebral column**, with the **diaphragm** dividing the thorax from the abdomen.

The sternum

The dagger-shaped **sternum** has three parts. The **manubrium**, with which the first and upper parts of the second costal cartilage and the clavicle articulate (Fig. 2a), lies at the level of the third and fourth thoracic vertebrae (see Fig. 1b). The lower parts of the second and third to seventh ribs articulate with the **body of the sternum** (level with T5–T8). The angle between the manubrium and body at the cartilaginous **manubriosternal joint** forms the **sternal angle (angle of Louis)** and this is a useful anatomical reference point. The small **xiphoid process** (xiphisternum) usually remains cartilaginous well into adult life.

The ribs and intercostal space

The first seven (**true or vertebrosternal**) of the 12 pairs of ribs are connected to the sternum by their costal cartilages. The hyaline cartilages of the eighth, ninth and tenth (**vertebrochondral**) ribs articulate with the cartilage above, and the eleventh and twelfth are free (**floating or vertebral ribs**). A typical rib (Fig. 2b) has a **head** with two **facets** for articulation with the corresponding vertebra, the intervertebral disc and the vertebra above. The rib also articulates at the **tubercle** with the transverse process of the corresponding vertebra. The two articular regions act like a hinge, forcing the rib to move through an axis passing through these areas. The flattened shaft of the rib is weakest at the **angle of the rib** and this is where it tends to fracture in an adult. The upper two ribs, protected by the clavicle and the two floating ribs, are least likely to fracture. There is a cervical rib attached to the transverse process of C7 in 0.5% of people and the presence of this rib may cause paraesthesiae or vascular problems, due to pressure on the brachial plexus or subclavian artery.

Intercostal spaces contain **external intercostal muscles** whose fibres pass downwards and forwards between the ribs, **internal intercostal muscles** whose fibres pass downwards and backwards and an incomplete **innermost intercostal layer** (Fig. 2c). They are innervated by **intercostal nerves**, which are the anterior primary rami of **thoracic nerves**. **Intercostal veins, arteries** and **nerves** lie in grooves on the undersurface of the corresponding rib, with the vein above, artery in the middle and nerve below.

The diaphragm

The dome-shaped **diaphragm** (Fig. 2d) separates the thorax and abdomen and consists of a muscular peripheral part and a **central tendon**, which is partly fused with the pericardium. The muscular diaphragm takes its origin from the vertebrae and arcuate ligaments, the rib cage and the sternum. The **right crus** arises from the upper three lumbar vertebrae and the **left crus** from the upper two lumbar vertebrae. Their fibrous medial borders form the **median arcuate ligament** over the front of the aorta. The **medial and lateral arcuate ligaments** are thickenings of the fascia overlying the **psoas major** and **quadratus lumborum**, respectively. The costal part of the diaphragm is attached to the inner aspects of the seventh to twelfth ribs and costal cartilages. The sternal part originates as two slips from the back of the xiphisternum. The **phrenic nerves (C3, 4, 5)** supply motor fibres. Sensory innervation of the central diaphragm also runs in the phrenic, and pain from irritation of the diaphragm is often referred to the corresponding dermatome for C4, the shoulder-tip. The lower intercostal nerves supply sensory fibres to the peripheral diaphragm. The aorta, thoracic duct and azygos vein pass through the diaphragm at the aortic opening at the level of T12. The oesophagus, branches of the left gastric artery and vein and both vagi pass through the oesophageal opening at the level of T10, and the inferior vena cava and right phrenic nerve pass through an opening at the level of T8.

Muscles of respiration

Inspiratory muscles all act to increase thoracic volume, causing intrapleural and alveolar pressure to fall to create an alveolar–mouth pressure gradient, drawing air into the lungs. The domes of the **diaphragm**, the main inspiratory muscle, move down when it contracts, by about 1.5 cm during quiet breathing and 6–7 cm during deep breathing. During quiet breathing, the first rib remains fairly still and the **external intercostals** elevate and evert the succeeding ribs, increasing both the anterior–posterior and transverse diameters of the chest wall, the so-called '**bucket-handle' action**. The expanded chest wall and lungs will recoil by themselves and quiet breathing uses no expiratory muscles.

When ventilation or resistance to breathing is increased, **accessory inspiratory muscles** aid inspiration. These include the **scalene muscles, sternomastoids** and **serratus anterior**. If the arms are fixed by grasping the edge of a table, contraction of the **pectoralis major**, which normally adducts the arm, helps expand the chest. When ventilation exceeds about 40 L/min, there is activation of expiratory muscles, especially **abdominal muscles (rectus abdominis, external and internal oblique)**, which speed up recoil of the diaphragm by raising intra-abdominal pressure.

In quiet breathing, ventilation is largely diaphragmatic, but when the phrenic nerves are damaged, normal ventilation can be maintained by the intercostal muscles. In a high cervical cord transection all respiratory muscles are paralysed, but when the damage is below the phrenic nerve roots (C3, 4, 5) breathing continues via the diaphragm alone. In the newborn, ribs are horizontal, so rib movements cannot increase the volume of the chest and breathing is entirely by the up-and-down action of the diaphragm or so-called **abdominal breathing**. As the ribs become more oblique with increasing age, the movement of the ribs becomes more important to give **thoracic breathing**.

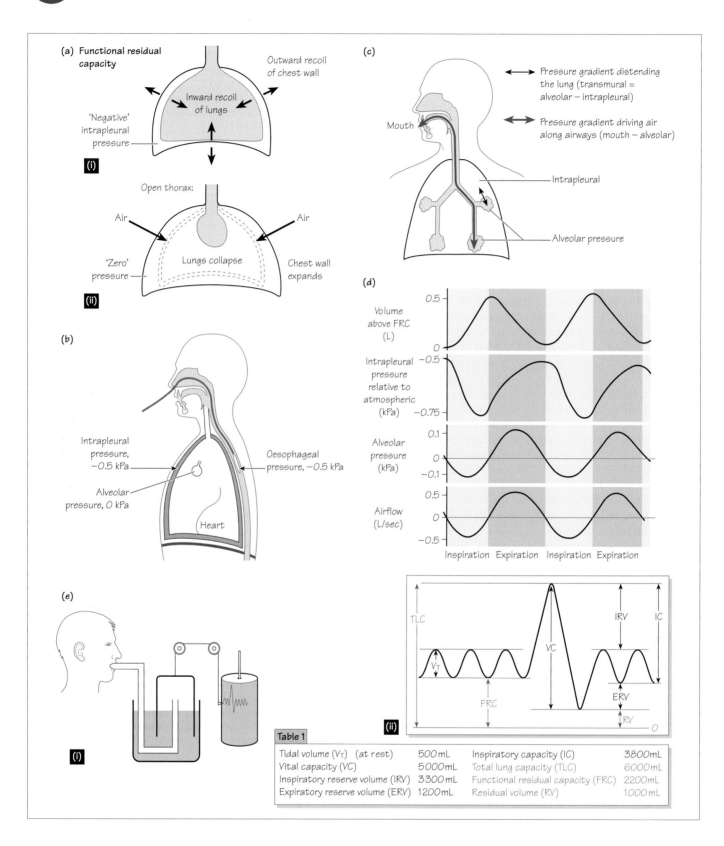

(a) Functional residual capacity

(i) Outward recoil of chest wall / Inward recoil of lungs / 'Negative' intrapleural pressure

(ii) Open thorax: Air / Lungs collapse / 'Zero' pressure / Chest wall expands

(b) Intrapleural pressure, −0.5 kPa / Oesophageal pressure, −0.5 kPa / Alveolar pressure, 0 kPa / Heart

(c) Mouth / Pressure gradient distending the lung (transmural = alveolar − intrapleural) / Pressure gradient driving air along airways (mouth − alveolar) / Intrapleural / Alveolar pressure

(d) Volume above FRC (L) / Intrapleural pressure relative to atmospheric (kPa) / Alveolar pressure (kPa) / Airflow (L/sec) / Inspiration Expiration Inspiration Expiration

(e) (i) / (ii) TLC / VC / V_T / FRC / IRV / IC / ERV / RV

Table 1

Tidal volume (V_T) (at rest)	500 mL	Inspiratory capacity (IC)	3800 mL
Vital capacity (VC)	5000 mL	Total lung capacity (TLC)	6000 mL
Inspiratory reserve volume (IRV)	3300 mL	Functional residual capacity (FRC)	2200 mL
Expiratory reserve volume (ERV)	1200 mL	Residual volume (RV)	1000 mL

Functional residual capacity

The volume left in the lungs at the end of a normal breath is known as the **functional residual capacity (FRC)**. At FRC, the respiratory muscles are relaxed and its volume is determined by the elastic properties of the lungs and chest wall.

The lungs are elastic bodies whose resting volume when removed from the body is very small. The natural resting position of the chest wall, seen when the chest is opened surgically, is about 1 L larger than at the end of a normal breath.

In the living respiratory system, the lungs are sealed within the chest wall. Between these two elastic structures is the **intrapleural space**, which contains only a few millilitres of fluid. When the respiratory muscles are relaxed the lungs and chest wall recoil in opposite directions, creating a subatmospheric ('negative') pressure in the space between them, and this tends to oppose the recoil of both the lungs and chest wall. **Functional residual capacity** occurs when the **outward recoil** of the chest wall exactly balances the **inward recoil** of the lungs (Fig. 3a). When the chest is opened, air enters the intrapleural space, the pressure becomes atmospheric and nothing opposes the recoil of the lungs and chest wall. The lungs shrink to a small volume and the chest wall springs out.

If the elastic recoil of either the lungs or chest wall is abnormally large or small, FRC will be abnormal. In lung fibrosis, the lungs are stiff and have increased elastic recoil, so the balance point, and hence FRC, occurs at a small lung volume. In emphysema, there is loss of alveolar tissue and with it, loss of elastic recoil. When the respiratory muscles are relaxed, the reduced elastic recoil of the lungs offers less opposition to the outward recoil of the chest wall and FRC is increased (the '**barrel chest**' of emphysema). Increased FRC can also occur because of 'air trapping' (see Chapter 7).

Intrapleural pressure

The space between the **visceral pleura** lining the lungs and the **parietal pleura** lining the chest wall is so small that measuring **intrapleural pressure** with a needle risks puncturing the lung. Intrapleural pressure can be indirectly assessed from **oesophageal pressure** (Fig. 3b). The oesophagus is normally closed at the top and bottom except during swallowing and in the upright subject the oesophageal pressure is the same as in the neighbouring intrapleural space. The subject swallows either a miniaturized pressure transducer or a balloon containing a little air connected by a tube to an external manometer. Gravity affects the fluid-lined intrapleural space and at FRC in an upright subject, the intrapleural pressure at the apex of the lungs is about $-0.5\,kPa$ ($-5\,cmH_2O$) and about $-0.2\,kPa$ ($-2\,cmH_2O$) at the bottom.

Pressures, flow and volume during a normal breathing cycle

During inspiration, the chest wall is expanded and intrapleural pressure falls. This increases the pressure gradient between the intrapleural space and alveoli (Fig. 3c), stretching the lungs. The alveoli expand and **alveolar pressure** falls, creating a pressure gradient between the mouth and alveoli, causing air to flow into the lungs. The airflow profile (Fig. 3d) closely follows that of alveolar pressure. During expiration, both intrapleural pressure and alveolar pressure rise. In quiet breathing, intrapleural pressure remains negative for the whole respiratory cycle, whereas alveolar pressure is negative during inspiration and positive during expiration. Alveolar pressure is always higher than intrapleural, because of the recoil of the lung. It is zero at the end of both inspiration and expiration and airflow ceases momentarily. When ventilation is increased, the changes of intrapleural and alveolar pressure are greater and in expiration intrapleural pressure may rise above atmospheric. In forced expiration, coughing or sneezing, intrapleural pressure may rise to $+8\,kPa$ ($+60\,mmHg$) or more.

Lung volumes

If a subject breathes in and out of a **simple water-filled spirometer** (Fig. 3e (i)), the drum falls and rises and the pen, attached by a pulley system, produces a trace (Fig. 3e (ii)) which illustrates the important lung volumes. Conventionally, volumes composed of two or more volumes are known as 'capacities', whereas those that cannot be subdivided are known as 'volumes'. The volume breathed in (or out) is known as the **tidal volume** and the trace shows several **resting tidal volumes**, which are typically about 500 mL. For the fourth breath, the subject breathes in and out as fully as possible. This maximum tidal volume is the **vital capacity** $(=V_T + IRV + ERV)$. At the end of a normal quiet inspiration, the subject could breathe in more and this is the **inspiratory reserve volume**. Similarly, the volume that he or she could exhale after a normal expiration is the **expiratory reserve volume**. At the end of a maximal breath out, the volume remaining in the lungs is the **residual volume**. **Functional residual capacity** and **total lung capacity** are the volumes in the lungs at the end of a normal expiration and after a maximal breath in, respectively. Typical values in an adult male are given in Table 1. Although a zero volume line is shown (Fig. 3e (ii)), it is not possible to know where this actually is on a trace, because the subject cannot empty the lungs into the drum. For this reason, although illustrated in Fig. 3e (ii), volumes shown in purple in Table 1 cannot be measured from a simple spirometer trace. They can be measured using **helium dilution** or **body plethysmography** (Chapter 20). The range of normal lung volumes is large and an individual's volumes must be assessed with the aid of **nomograms** that give the predicted value of each volume for the subject's age, sex and height.

(a) Standard respiratory symbols

Primary symbols

F = Fractional concentration of gas   P = Pressure or partial pressure
C = Content of a gas in blood   S = Saturation of haemoglobin with oxygen
V = Volume of a gas   Q = Volume of blood

A dot over a letter means a time derivative, e.g. $\dot{V}$ = Ventilation (L/min)
$\dot{Q}$ = Blood flow (L/min)

Secondary symbols

Gas: I = Inspired gas   **Blood:** a = Arterial
     E = Expired gas   v = Venous
     A = Alveolar gas   c = Capillary
     D = Dead space gas   A dash means mixed or mean
     T = Tidal   e.g. $\bar{v}$ = Mixed venous
     B = Barometric   A ' after a symbol means end
    ET = End-tidal   e.g. c' = End-capillary

Tertiary symbols   Examples

O_2 = Oxygen $\dot{V}O_2$ = Oxygen consumption
CO_2 = Carbon dioxide P_ACO_2 = Alveolar partial pressure
CO = Carbon monoxide   of carbon dioxide

(b) Correction factors for gas volumes

$$\text{Volume}_{(BTPS)} = \text{volume}_{(ATPS)} \left(\frac{273 + 37}{273 + t^0C}\right)\left(\frac{P_B - P_{H_2O}}{P_B - 6.3^*}\right) \quad *47 \text{ if } P_B \text{ and } P_{H_2O} \text{ are in mmHg}$$

$$\text{Volume}_{(STPD)} = \text{volume}_{(ATPS)} \left(\frac{273}{273 + t^0C}\right)\left(\frac{P_B - P_{H_2O}}{101^*}\right) \quad *760 \text{ if } P_B \text{ and } P_{H_2O} \text{ are in mmHg}$$

(c) Partial pressure of a gas in a liquid

Gas phase, Pg

Liquid phase liquid X, PXg

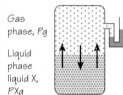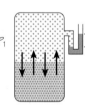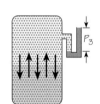

Gas phase, Pg

Liquid phase liquid Y, PYg

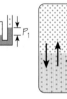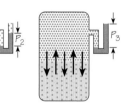

Liquid X containing dissolved gas, g, is exposed to a gas phase containing g at three different partial pressures, P_1, P_2, P_3. Only when the Pg = P_2 does the number of gas molecules leaving the liquid per minute (↑) equal the number entering the liquid (↓) – i.e. the liquid and gas phases are in equilibrium.

∴ Partial pressure of gas, g, in liquid X (PXg) = P_2

Liquid Y also contains gas, g and is also in equilibrium with the gas phase when Pg = P_2

∴ Partial pressure of gas, g, in liquid Y (PYg) = P_2

However, the solubility of gas, g, in liquid Y is less than in liquid X, so at the same partial pressure, liquid Y contains a lower concentration of g.

Note: In the bottom left flask, gas moves against its concentration gradient.

To understand the processes involved in respiration and how valid measurements are made, it is important to understand the behaviour of gases in both gas mixtures and in liquids.

Fractional concentration and partial pressure of gases in a gas mixture

Dalton's law states that when two or more gases, which do not react chemically, are present in the same container, the total pressure is the sum of the partial pressures (the pressure that each gas would exert if isolated in the container).

The total pressure exerted by the atmosphere was traditionally measured by inverting a long mercury-filled glass tube over a mercury reservoir. At sea level, the height of the column supported is normally about 760 mm, so barometric pressure is 760 mmHg (torr), which in SI units is about 101 kPa (1 kPa = 7.50 mmHg). Dried air contains 21% oxygen. The remaining gases are nitrogen, 78.1%, and inert gases such as argon and helium, 0.9%, although for convenience these physiologically inert gases are often pooled as 'nitrogen, 79%'. Air is considered to be CO_2-free, as the amount present (0.04%) is very small. Standardized symbols used in respiratory physiology are shown in Fig. 4a.

According to Dalton's law:

Dry partial pressure oxygen in inspired air (PIO_2)
= oxygen fraction (FO_2) × total barometric pressure (PB)
= 0.21 × 101 (760) = 21.2 kPa (159 mmHg)

At **altitude**, the oxygen fraction of air is unaltered but barometric pressure is reduced, being about 33.6 kPa (252 mmHg) on the top of Everest.

Water vapour pressure

Air contains variable amounts of water vapour, depending on the water it has been exposed to and the temperature. The maximum or **saturated water vapour pressure** is higher in warm than cool air: at 20°C, it is 2.33 kPa (17.5 mmHg), whereas at body temperature (37°C), it is 6.3 kPa (47 mmHg). The **relative humidity** (actual/saturated water vapour pressure × 100%) of inspired air varies with climate; if it is 40% at 20°C, water vapour pressure will be 0.9 kPa (7 mmHg). The presence of water vapour means that ambient FO_2 and FN_2 are usually a little lower than the dry fractions given above. Air passing down the airways quickly reaches body temperature (37°C) and 100% saturation. Total pressure remains close to barometric, so the added water vapour causes significant dilution of the other gases. The available pressure for the other gases is therefore PB −6.3 kPa (PB −47 mmHg).

The **partial pressure of moist inspired oxygen (PIO_2)** = 0.21 × (PB − saturated vapour pressure at 37°C). At sea level, this is 19.9 kPa (=0.21 × (101−6.3)) or 149.7 mmHg. At altitude, as PB falls, the dilution of inspired gas with water vapour becomes relatively more important. On the top of Everest, where PB is about 33.6 kPa (252 mmHg), moist PIO_2 is 5.7 kPa (43 mmHg).

The effect of pressure and temperature on gas volumes

The inverse relationship between the volume of a perfect gas and its pressure, described by **Boyle's law ($P \propto 1/V$)** and the direct relationship between volume and absolute temperature (=273 +°C) described by **Charles' law ($V \propto T$)** are important when measuring gas volumes. Expired gas collected in a bag or spirometer will shrink, both because of the direct effect of falling temperature (Charles' law) and because water vapour condenses as temperature falls. To enable valid comparisons, volumes at **ambient temperature and pressure saturated with water (ATPS)** are corrected to those they would occupy under standard conditions. For measurements of lung volumes, this is to **body temperature and pressure saturated with water (BTPS)**. For O_2 consumption or CO_2 production, **standard temperature and pressure dry (STPD)** (0°C, 101.3 kPa (760 mmHg), $PH_2O = 0$) are usually used, so that each litre contains the same number of molecules (1 mole ≈ 22.4 L).

Boyle's law, Charles' law and the reduction of saturated vapour pressure with temperature are combined in the equations for correcting volumes given in Fig. 4b.

Gases dissolved in liquids

If a gas is exposed to a liquid to which it does not react, gas particles will move into the liquid. **Henry's law** states that the number of molecules dissolving in the liquid is directly proportional to the partial pressure at the surface of the gas.

The constant of proportionality is the solubility of the gas in the liquid and it is affected by the gas, the liquid and the temperature, tending to fall as temperature rises.

Content of dissolved gas X in a liquid Y
= solubility of X in Y × partial pressure of X at surface

The **partial pressure of a gas in a liquid** or **gas tension** is a more difficult concept than that of partial pressure in a gas phase, where we can visualize the pressure of the molecules holding up a column of mercury. The molecules of the gas in the liquid phase will move about in the liquid and have a tendency to escape from the surface, which can be opposed by molecules of the same gas in a gas phase in contact with the liquid (Fig. 4c). If the partial pressure of the gas in the gas phase is altered until there is no net movement of gas between the gas phase and the liquid phase, the gas and liquid are said to be in equilibrium. By definition, the partial pressure of a gas in a liquid is equal to the partial pressure of that gas in a gas phase with which it is in equilibrium. Partial pressure gradient (not concentration gradient) always determines the direction of movement between phases such as a gas and liquid phase.

Note on time derivative symbols

Time derivatives are properly denoted by a dot over the symbol (e.g. $\dot{V}_A$, alveolar ventilation in L/min, see Fig. 4a). However, for terms such as the ventilation/perfusion ratio (V_A/Q) the dots are often omitted, and this convention is followed throughout this book.

5 Diffusion

(a) The alveolar–capillary membrane

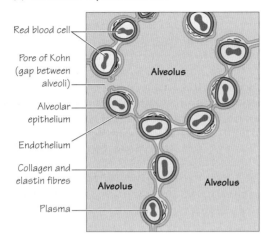

- Red blood cell
- Pore of Kohn (gap between alveoli)
- Alveolar epithelium
- Endothelium
- Collagen and elastin fibres
- Plasma

Alveolus

Alveolus   Alveolus

(b) Transfer of gases across alveolar–capillary membrane

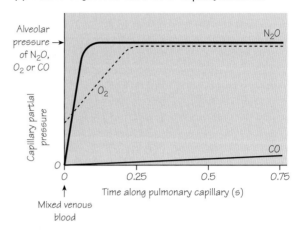

Alveolar pressure of N_2O, O_2 or CO

Capillary partial pressure

N_2O

O_2

CO

Mixed venous blood

Time along pulmonary capillary (s)

0   0.25   0.5   0.75

(c) Diffusion through a sheet of tissue

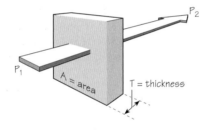

P_2

P_1

A = area

T = thickness

(e) The oxygen cascade: oxygen tension from ambient air to mitochondria

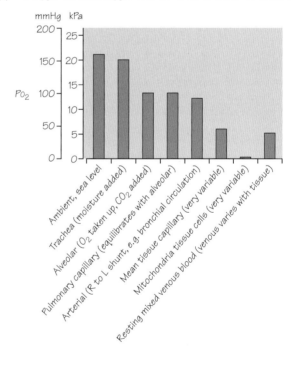

mmHg   kPa

PO_2

200   25
150   20
100   15
50   10
       5
0   0

- Ambient, sea level
- Trachea (moisture added)
- Alveolar (O_2 taken up, CO_2 added)
- Pulmonary capillary (equilibrates with alveolar)
- Arterial (R to L shunt, e.g. bronchial circulation)
- Mean tissue capillary (very variable)
- Mitochondria tissue cells (very variable)
- Resting mixed venous blood (venous varies with tissue)

(d) The diffusion path through the alveolar–capillary membrane

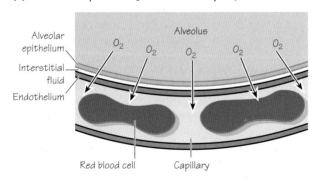

Alveolus

- Alveolar epithelium
- Interstitial fluid
- Endothelium

O_2 O_2 O_2 O_2 O_2

Red blood cell   Capillary

Oxygen and carbon dioxide are transported in the body by a mixture of **bulk flow** and **diffusion**. Bulk flow, generated by differences in total fluid pressure, is important in most of the airways and in transporting blood containing these gases between pulmonary and tissue capillaries. Diffusion, driven by partial pressure differences, is important in the last few millimetres of the airways, across the alveolar–capillary membrane and between tissue capillaries and mitochondria.

The alveolar–capillary membrane (Fig. 5a)

Adult male lungs contain about 300 million alveoli, approximately 0.2 mm in diameter. Between neighbouring alveoli are two layers of **alveolar epithelium** each resting on a basement membrane, enclosing the interstitial space, containing **pulmonary capillaries**, **elastin** and **collagen fibres**. The **alveolar epithelium** and **capillary endothelium** form the **alveolar–capillary membrane**, through which gases diffuse. It is very thin (<0.4 µm), except where collagen and elastin fibres are concentrated, with a total surface area of about 85 m². There are two types of alveolar epithelial cell. **Type I cells** line the alveoli and are relatively devoid of organelles. The round **type II cells** have large nuclei, microvilli and contain striated osmiophilic lamellar bodies storing surfactant, an important component of alveolar lining fluid (Chapter 6).

Diffusion and perfusion limitation (Fig. 5b)

If gas containing the poorly soluble gas nitrous oxide (N_2O) is inhaled, pulmonary capillary P_{N_2O} rises and quickly equilibrates with alveolar P_{N_2O}. With no alveolar–capillary partial pressure gradient remaining, diffusion ceases along the rest of the pulmonary capillary and uptake can only be increased by increasing pulmonary capillary blood flow. N_2O uptake is said to be **perfusion-limited**. In contrast, when breathing a carbon monoxide (CO) containing mixture, the CO combines so avidly with haemoglobin that pulmonary capillary P_{CO} rises little. The pressure gradient driving diffusion is preserved along the capillary and CO uptake would not be increased by increased perfusion. Improved ease of diffusion, with reduced thickness or increased area of the alveolar–capillary membrane, would increase CO uptake. CO transfer is **diffusion-limited**. Oxygen transfer lies between these two extremes, but is normally perfusion-limited.

Factors affecting diffusion across a membrane (Fick and Graham's laws)

For a sheet of tissue of area A and thickness T through which gas g is passing (Fig. 5c):

$$\text{Rate of transfer of gas } g \propto \frac{A}{T}(P_1 - P_2)$$

The constant of proportionality

$$= \frac{\text{Solubility of the gas in the membrane(s)}}{\sqrt{\text{Molecular weight of the gas}}}$$

Although the molecular weight of CO_2 is about 1.4 times that of O_2, it is about 20 times more soluble, and so diffuses more easily.

For the alveolar–capillary membrane, the pressure gradient driving diffusion is alveolar (P_A) minus mean pulmonary capillary ($P_{\bar{c}}$). The constants (s, mw, A and T) can be combined to give a single constant, the **diffusing capacity** ($D_L g$) of the lungs for gas, g:

$$\text{Rate of transfer of gas, } g = D_L g (P_A - P_{\bar{c}})$$

Oxygen diffusing capacity, D_{LO_2}

$$= \frac{\text{Oxygen uptake from the lungs } (\dot{V}_{O_2})}{P_{A}O_2 - P_{\bar{c}}O_2}$$

Although measurement of D_{LO_2} is desirable, it is not possible because mean capillary P_{O_2} ($P_{\bar{c}O_2}$) cannot be measured.

CO diffuses through the same pathway as O_2 and its rate of diffusion is affected by the same factors that affect oxygen transfer. However, unlike D_{LO_2}, D_{LCO} is measurable. Once CO arrives in the pulmonary capillary blood, it too combines with haemoglobin. Haemoglobin has approximately 240 times the affinity for CO than it does for O_2 and consequently as CO is transferred, almost all of it enters chemical combination and the mean pulmonary capillary P_{CO} can be assumed to be zero.

This simplifies the equation to:

$$D_{L}CO = \frac{\text{Carbon monoxide uptake from the lungs } (\dot{V}_{CO})}{P_{A}CO}$$

Several methods are used for measuring $D_{L}CO$, but all involve breathing a low level of CO (e.g. 0.3%). Helium is included as a measure of dilution by alveolar gas. By sampling exhaled gas, CO uptake and mean alveolar P_{CO} can be calculated. The normal value depends on the method used, but is about 15–30 mL/min/mmHg (112–225 mL/min/kPa). $D_{L}CO$ is divided by alveolar volume to give an index (K_{CO}) that corrects for different lung volumes. As both D_{LO_2} and $D_{L}CO$ are affected by the rate of gas combination with haemoglobin in addition to factors affecting diffusion, some prefer the alternative term transfer factor (T_{LO_2} and $T_{L}CO$).

Factors affecting D_LCO (T_LCO)

$D_{L}CO$ is lowered by reduced alveolar–capillary membrane area in emphysema, pulmonary emboli or lung resection and by increased thickness in pulmonary oedema. In pulmonary fibrosis the alveolar–capillary membrane is both thickened and reduced in area giving a low $D_{L}CO$ with a less affected K_{CO}. Increased pulmonary blood volume in exercise increases the effective area increasing $D_{L}CO$. $D_{L}CO$ is increased with polycythaemia and reduced in anaemia. $D_{L}CO$ is therefore non-specific but it is sensitive and may reveal abnormalities when other lung function tests are normal. Hypoventilation does not affect $D_{L}CO$ because the reduced CO uptake is caused by reduced $P_{A}CO$.

The oxygen cascade (Fig. 5e) shows how P_{O_2} falls between air and mitochondria. Mitochondrial oxidative phosphorylation will cease when P_{O_2} falls below 1 mmHg (0.13 kPa) and this ultimately limits the capillary P_{O_2} that can be tolerated and therefore the amount of oxygen that can be removed as blood passes through the tissues. Capillary P_{O_2} must remain high enough to drive diffusion to cells at a rate sufficient to match oxygen consumption and maintain mitochondrial P_{O_2} above this critical level.

6 Lung mechanics: elastic forces

(a) Static pressure–volume loop

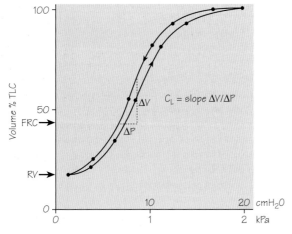

C_L = slope $\Delta V/\Delta P$

Transmural pressure (= – intrapleural pressure
since measurements taken at zero airflow)

RV = Residual volume	FRC = Functional residual capacity
TLC = Total lung capacity	C_L = Lung compliance

(b) Dynamic pressure–volume loop

If intrapleural pressure and volume are recorded continuously
(lower panel) a pressure–volume loop (upper panel) can be
constructed from pairs of simultaneous measurements of volume
e.g. (b) with pressure (b'). Alternatively the pressure and volume
signals can be fed into an X-Y plotter.

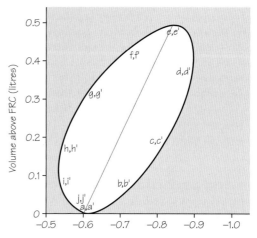

Intrapleural pressure relative to atmospheric (kPa)

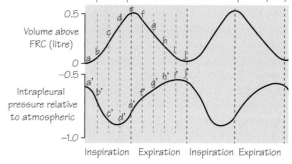

Inspiration   Expiration   Inspiration   Expiration

(c) Surface tension

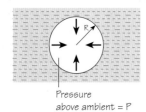

Pressure
above ambient = P

Laplace's equation

$$P = \frac{2T}{R}$$

T = Surface tension

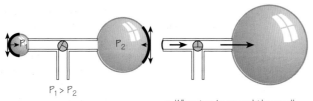

$P_1 > P_2$

∴ When tap is opened the small
bubble empties into the large

(d) Effect of surface area

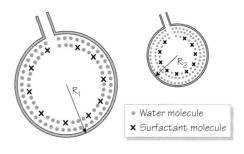

• Water molecule
✕ Surfactant molecule

$R_2 < R_1$ but $T_2 < T_1$ because surface concentration of surfactant
is higher when the alveolus is small
The fall in R is more than offset by the fall in T,
∴ since $P = \frac{2T}{R}$, P does not rise, but falls as the alveolus shrinks

To breathe in, the inspiratory muscles must contract to overcome the impedance offered by the lungs and chest wall. This is mainly in the form of frictional **airway resistance** (Chapter 7) and **elastic resistance** to stretching of the lung and chest wall tissues and the fluid lining the alveoli.

Assessing the stiffness of the lungs: lung compliance

The 'stretchiness' of the lung is usually assessed as lung compliance (C_L), which is the change in lung volume per unit change in distending pressure ($C_L = \Delta V/\Delta P$). The distending pressure, P, is the pressure difference across the lung, which equals alveolar − intrapleural pressure.

Intrapleural pressure can be assessed using an oesophageal balloon (Chapter 3). Alveolar pressure cannot easily be measured directly, but when no air is flowing alveolar pressure must equal mouth pressure (i.e. zero). The transmural pressure, P, is then equal to −intrapleural pressure. The subject breathes in steps and measurements are taken while the breath is held and plotted as a **static pressure–volume (P–V) curve** (Fig. 6a). The curve flattens as the lung volume approaches total lung capacity. The inspiratory curve is slightly different from the expiratory curve and this **hysteresis** is a common property of elastic bodies. **Static lung compliance** is the slope of the steepest part of this static pressure–volume curve in the region just above functional residual capacity (FRC).

Lung compliance is normally about 1.5 L/kPa, but as with lung volumes it is affected by the subject's size, age and gender. In **restrictive disease**, such as lung fibrosis, lung compliance is low. Like a stiff spring, once stretched, fibrosed lungs have an increased tendency to shrink back to their resting position or increased **elastic recoil**. The loss of alveolar tissue in **emphysema** makes them easier to stretch and lung compliance is increased. Although safe, swallowing an oesophageal balloon is not very pleasant or convenient. Fortunately, it is often possible to deduce that a patient has stiff lungs from other measurements such as **total lung capacity (TLC)**, **FRC** (Chapters 3, 20 & 29), forced expiratory volume in 1 second (**FEV$_1$**) and forced vital capacity (**FVC**) (Chapter 20).

Dynamic pressure–volume loops and dynamic compliance

A **dynamic pressure–volume loop** (upper panel of Fig. 6b) is obtained from continuous measurements of intrapleural pressure and volume during a normal breathing cycle (lower panel of Fig. 6b). There are two points, at the ends of inspiration and expiration, where airflow and alveolar pressure are zero (a, a′ and e, e′) and the slope of the line joining these points is **dynamic compliance**. In health, its value is similar to the **static compliance**, but in some diseases it may be lower, as stiff areas may fill preferentially during normal breathing. Between the two zero flow points, the dynamic P–V loop appears fatter than the static P–V loop, as intrapleural pressure must change more to drive airflow. In fact, the area of the dynamic loop is a measure of the work done against airway resistance (Chapter 7).

The air–fluid interface lining the alveoli

During inspiration, as well as stretching the collagen and elastin fibres, the **surface tension** forces at the air–alveolar lining fluid interface must be overcome. At the surface of a bubble, the attraction of the fluid molecules for each other creates a tension, which tends to shrink the bubble (Fig. 6c). Laplace discovered that a gas bubble in a liquid would shrink until the pressure, P, within it reached a value of 2T/R, where T is a constant, the surface tension of the fluid and R is the radius of the bubble. When a bubble has air on both sides there are two air–fluid interfaces and P = 4T/R. The **law of Laplace (P = 2T/R or 4T/R)** predicts that if two bubbles are made of the same fluid, the smaller bubble will have a higher pressure within it—since when the radius of curvature is small, a greater proportion of the surface tension is directed to the centre of the bubble (lower panel of Fig. 6.1c). When the two bubbles are connected, the small bubble empties into the large bubble as air flows down the pressure gradient.

The presence of an air–fluid interface creates several potential problems:
1 It reduces lung compliance and the higher the surface tension the lower the compliance.
2 The alveoli would be inherently unstable, with the smaller alveoli tending to collapse completely.
3 As the fluid tends to shrink away from the alveolar cells, it would create a suction force tending to cause **transudation** of fluid from the nearby pulmonary capillaries.

The absence of these problems in normal adults is thought to be partly due to the presence in the alveolar lining fluid of **surfactant**.

Surfactant

Pulmonary surfactant is a mixture of **phospholipids**, such phosphatidylcholine and proteins, produced by the **type II alveolar cells** (Chapter 5). The presence of these substances in the **alveolar lining fluid** lowers the surface tension and increases compliance. The phospholipids have a **hydrophilic** end that lies in the alveolar fluid and a **hydrophobic** end that projects into the alveolar gas and as a result they float on the surface of the lining fluid. As an alveolus shrinks, its surface area diminishes and the surface concentration of surfactant rises (Fig. 6d). As surface tension falls with increasing surface concentration of surfactant, the increased tendency for alveoli to collapse when they shrink is offset and stability improved. Alveolar stability is also aided by the connection and mutual pull of neighbouring alveoli, a phenomenon known as **alveolar interdependence**.

Surfactant production in the fetus gradually increases in the last third of pregnancy and may be inadequate in babies born prematurely, giving rise to the typical problems of **neonatal respiratory distress syndrome (NRDS)**—stiff lungs and areas of collapse (Chapters 16 & 17).

Surfactant proteins (e.g. SP-A, SP-B, SP-C and SP-D) contribute to the surface tension lowering actions of phospholipids, as well as having other functions such as host defence. They are probably the reason why natural surfactants have proved more effective for treating NRDS than artificial surfactant composed only of phospholipids.

Lung mechanics: airway resistance

(a) Laminar and turbulent flow

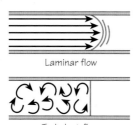

Laminar flow

Turbulent flow

(b) Main factors influencing bronchomotor tone

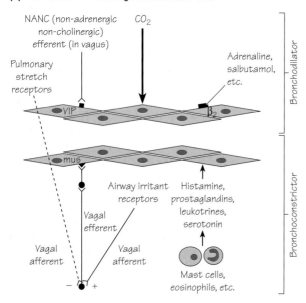

NANC (non-adrenergic non-cholinergic) efferent (in vagus)

CO_2

Pulmonary stretch receptors

Adrenaline, salbutamol, etc.

Bronchodilator

VIP

β_2

mus

Airway irritant receptors

Histamine, prostaglandins, leukotrines, serotonin

Vagal efferent

Vagal efferent

Vagal afferent

Vagal afferent

Mast cells, eosinophils, etc.

Bronchoconstrictor

$\beta_2 = \beta_2$ adrenergic receptor, VIP = vasoactive intestinal peptide receptor, mus = muscuranic cholinergic receptor

(d) Dynamic compression of airways

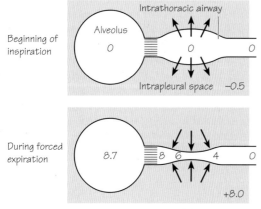

Beginning of inspiration

Alveolus
0

Intrathoracic airway

0   0

Intrapleural space   −0.5

During forced expiration

8.7

8   6   4   0

+8.0

Numbers are pressures in kPa (1 kPa = 7.5 mmHg)

(c) The effect of effort on inspiratory and expiratory airflow

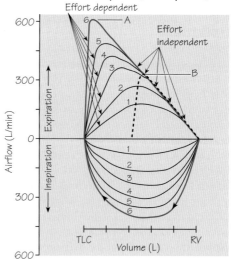

Effort dependent

Effort independent

Airflow (L/min)

Expiration

Inspiration

TLC   Volume (L)   RV

- - - = Flow–volume curve for maximum effort from partly filled lungs
A = Peak expiratory flow rate with lungs filled to total lung capacity
B = Peak expiratory flow rate for partly filled lungs filled (RV + 3 litre)
TLC = Total lung capacity, RV = Residual volume

(e) Maximum flow–volume loops

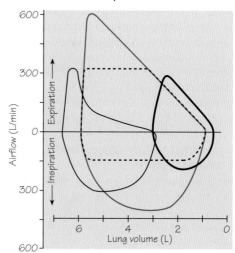

Airflow (L/min)

Expiration

Inspiration

Lung volume (L)

—— Normal curve

—— Obstructive airway disease of smaller airways. Note:
- concave appearance of forced expiratory curve
- forced inspiratory flow affected less than forced expiratory flow

- - - Upper airway obstruction (e.g. tracheal stenosis). Note:
- flat topped flow–volume curve
- forced inspiratory flow affected as much as expiratory flow

—— Restrictive lung disease. Low peak flow rates are related to low volume. (Note: this figure is drawn to show the relationship between these traces by using absolute lung volume which cannot actually be obtained from a flow–volume loop alone).

Airflow is driven by the mouth–alveolar pressure gradient generated by the respiratory muscles (Chapters 2 and 3).

$$\text{Airflow} = \frac{\Delta P \; (= \text{mouth} - \text{alveolar pressure})}{\text{RAW} \; (= \text{resistance of the airways})}$$

In **laminar flow**, gas particles move parallel to the walls, with centre layers moving faster than outer ones, creating a cone-shaped front (Fig. 7a). The factors affecting laminar flow of a fluid of viscosity, η, in smooth straight tubes of length, ℓ, and radius, r, are described in **Poiseuille's equation**:

$$\text{Flow} = \frac{\Delta P}{R} = \Delta P \frac{\pi r^4}{8 \ell \eta} \qquad \therefore R = \frac{8 \ell \eta}{\pi r^4}$$

Halving the radius of an airway increases its resistance 16-fold. However, although the resistance of an individual bronchiole is high, there are thousands in parallel. The total resistance of each generation of peripheral airways is normally low and the overall resistance of lung airways is dominated by the larger airways. Outside the lung, the nose and pharynx contribute substantial resistance, which can be reduced by mouth breathing, for example, during exercise. Peripheral airways are often affected by disease, but because their resistance must increase considerably to measurably affect airway resistance (RAW) they are known as the **silent zone**.

At higher linear velocities, especially in wide airways and near branch points, flow may become **turbulent**. With turbulence, the wave front is square and flow $\propto \sqrt{\Delta P}$ (not ΔP), reflecting the dissipation of energy in the formation of eddies. Normally, at rest, flow is laminar throughout the airways, but in exercise it may become turbulent, especially in the trachea, generating characteristic harsh breath sounds.

Factors affecting airway resistance
Bronchial smooth muscle and epithelium
Bronchial smooth muscle (Fig. 7b) receives a **parasympathetic bronchoconstrictor** nerve supply, which forms the efferent limb of a reflex from airway irritant receptors. The airways contain β_2-adrenergic receptors, which cause relaxation when stimulated by circulating **epinephrine** (adrenaline) or drugs such as salbutamol. Sympathetic innervation of the airways is sparse in humans. Parasympathetic bronchoconstriction is inhibited by activation of airway stretch receptors and CO_2 has a direct bronchodilator effect. Pollutants (e.g. sulphur dioxide, ozone) and substances released from mast cells and eosinophils can increase RAW via bronchoconstriction, mucosal oedema, mucus hypersecretion, mucus plugging and epithelial shedding, all of which are important in asthma (Chapter 23). Airway resistance can also be increased by chronic mucosal hypertrophy in chronic obstructive pulmonary disease (COPD) (Chapter 25) and by material within the airways, such as inhaled foreign bodies or tumours (Chapter 39).

Transmural (airway – intrapleural) pressure gradient
The pressure difference across airways can have important effects on their calibre, and this underlies the effects of effort on airflow illustrated in Fig. 7c. Airflow is measured continuously and plotted against lung volume as the subject breathes between residual volume (RV) and total lung capacity (TLC). The inspiratory airflow at any volume increases progressively with increasing effort (1 = minimum effort, 6 = maximum effort). The flow–volume curves for progressively increasing expiratory efforts (upper traces 1–6) are more complicated. In the early part of expiration from TLC, flow is **effort-dependent**, but towards the end of the breath, as volume declines, the traces produced at different effort levels come together. Expiratory airflow towards the end of a breath is **effort-independent** and determined by lung volume. **Peak expiratory flow rate** (PEFR) is seen to be reduced (B in Fig. 7c) if the lungs are only partially filled at the start of the forced expiration.

Effort-independent airflow is explained by **dynamic compression of airways**. Before the start of inspiration (Fig. 7d, upper panel) pressure along the airways is zero, intrapleural pressure is negative (Chapter 3) and transmural pressure acts to hold airways open. Intrapleural pressure is negative during both quiet and forced inspiration and it remains negative in quiet expiration, so transmural pressure holds airways open. In a forced expiration, however, expiratory muscle contraction raises intrapleural pressure well above atmospheric (e.g. 8 kPa, 60 mmHg), increasing the pressure gradient from alveoli to mouth. This would be expected to increase airflow, but the increased intrapleural pressure also acts to compress airways. Airway pressure falls progressively along the airway and at some point—usually in the bronchi—the airway pressure will be sufficiently below intrapleural pressure for the airway to collapse, despite its cartilaginous support. Pressure will then build up distally, opening the airways again. The resulting fluttering walls can be seen on bronchoscopy and produce the brassy note audible on forced expiration in normal people.

RAW in disease
Increased airway resistance is important in many diseases and can be measured using a body plethysmograph. In healthy individuals, RAW is about 0.2 kPa/L/s (1.5 mmHg/L/s). More commonly, airway resistance is assessed indirectly from forced expiratory measurements, such as **forced expiratory volume in 1 second** (FEV_1), **forced vital capacity** (FVC) and PEFR (Chapter 20). Especially useful is the **forced expiratory ratio** (FER = FEV_1/FVC), which is reduced when RAW is increased in **obstructive pulmonary disease**. High airway resistance accentuates dynamic compression of airways by augmenting the pressure drop along airways. In addition, the airways may be less able to resist compression, in emphysema because of reduced radial traction and in asthma because of bronchoconstriction. Collapse of small airways may occur, leading to incomplete expiration, **air trapping** and increased functional residual capacity. Inability to produce high expiratory airflow impairs effective coughing, which can lead to a vicious cycle as secretions accumulate, further increasing RAW and further reducing peak flow.

Expiratory wheezes (rhonchi), heard in asthma and other obstructive diseases, are probably generated by oscillations in opposing airway walls near their point of closure, like sounds from the reeds of an oboe. A reasonable airflow is needed to generate such sounds and when constriction becomes very severe, they disappear to give the ominous silent chest seen in life-threatening asthma. Small airway collapse leads to characteristic shape of the maximum flow–volume curve in obstructive airway disease (Fig. 7e), which differs from that in upper airway obstruction and restrictive lung disease.

8 Carriage of oxygen

(a) Haemoglobin structure

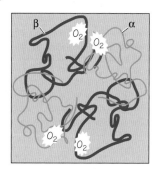

Haemoglobin is composed of four subunits, each containing a protein chain (globin) and a haem group. Normal adult haemoglobin, HbA, contains two identical α-chains composed of 141 amino acids and two β-chains composed of 146 amino acids. The haem group (◯) is attached to each chain at a histidine residue and each has an iron atom in the ferrous form, which binds to an oxygen molecule. The haem groups lie in crevices in the crumpled ball of globin chains. The exact 3D (or quaternary) structure of haemoglobin can change and alter the accessibility of the oxygen binding site. Each molecule of haemoglobin can bind up to four molecules of oxygen in a series of reactions which can be summarized as:

$$Hb_4 + 4O_2 \Leftrightarrow Hb_4(O_2)_4$$

(b) The oxygen–haemoglobin dissociation curve, haemoglobin concentration, 15 g/dL

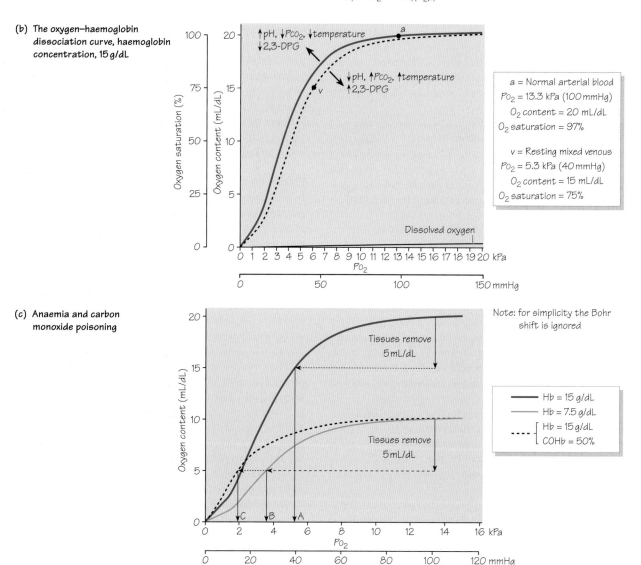

↑pH, ↓P_{CO_2}, ↓temperature
↓2,3-DPG

↓pH, ↑P_{CO_2}, ↑temperature
↑2,3-DPG

Dissolved oxygen

a = Normal arterial blood
P_{O_2} = 13.3 kPa (100 mmHg)
O_2 content = 20 mL/dL
O_2 saturation = 97%

v = Resting mixed venous
P_{O_2} = 5.3 kPa (40 mmHg)
O_2 content = 15 mL/dL
O_2 saturation = 75%

(c) Anaemia and carbon monoxide poisoning

Note: for simplicity the Bohr shift is ignored

Tissues remove 5 mL/dL

Tissues remove 5 mL/dL

	Hb = 15 g/dL
	Hb = 7.5 g/dL
	Hb = 15 g/dL COHb = 50%

At rest, an adult male consumes about 250 mL oxygen/min, which may rise to more than 4000 mL/min in exercise if he is very fit. Oxygen diffuses from alveolus to blood until equilibrium is reached when pulmonary capillary P_{O_2} equals alveolar P_{O_2}. The **solubility** of oxygen in blood is low—0.000225 mL oxygen per mL of blood per kPa (0.00003 mL/mL/mmHg)—so that at a normal arterial P_{O_2} of 13.3 kPa (100 mmHg) there is only 0.3 mL dissolved in each 100 mL of blood. The main function of the red blood cell pigment, **haemoglobin**, whose structure is shown in Fig. 8a, is to carry the large quantities of oxygen needed by the tissues.

Each gram of haemoglobin combines with up to 1.34 mL oxygen, so with a haemoglobin concentration, [Hb], of 15 g/dL, blood contains a maximum of 20 mL/dL oxygen bound to haemoglobin. This is known as the **oxygen capacity**, which varies with [Hb]. The actual amount of oxygen bound also depends on the P_{O_2}. The percentage of the available binding sites bound to oxygen is known as the **oxygen saturation**.

Oxygen saturation:

$$\frac{\text{Amount of oxygen bound to haemoglobin, mL/dL}}{\text{oxygen capacity, mL/dL}} \times 100\%$$

The oxygen content of the blood (mL/dL) equals the sum of haemoglobin-bound oxygen and the small amount of dissolved oxygen. The rate of rise of oxygen content with increasing partial pressure depends on the number of free haemoglobin binding sites remaining and their affinity for oxygen. As each oxygen molecule binds in turn to the four haem groups, the quaternary structure alters and the affinity of the remaining binding sites for oxygen increases. This **cooperative binding** increases the steepness of the **oxygen–haemoglobin dissociation curve** in the middle (Fig. 8b), but the curve flattens again at partial pressures above about 8 kPa (60 mmHg) because there are few unfilled binding sites remaining. In arterial blood, P_{O_2} is normally about 13 kPa (100 mmHg), oxygen saturation about 97%, and, with a normal [Hb], an oxygen content of about 20 mL/dL. Rises or modest falls in P_{O_2} from 13 kPa (100 mmHg), for example during hyperventilation or mild hypoventilation, cause little change in the arterial oxygen content, as the dissociation curve is flat in this region. More severe reductions in P_{O_2}, to levels in the steep region, are associated with significant reductions in oxygen saturation and content. Consequently, breathing oxygen-enriched air may significantly raise arterial oxygen content and hence exercise capacity at altitude and in patients with chronic hypoxic respiratory disease, but has little effect on a normal person at sea level.

Low P_{O_2} in tissue capillaries causes oxygen release from haemoglobin, whereas the high P_{O_2} in pulmonary capillaries causes oxygen binding. The affinity of haemoglobin for oxygen and hence position of the dissociation curve varies with local conditions. A reduced oxygen affinity, shown by a right shift in the curve, is caused by a fall in pH, a rise in P_{CO_2} (the **Bohr effect**) or increased temperature (Fig. 8b). These changes occur in metabolically active tissues such as exercising muscle and encourage oxygen release. In the lungs, oxygen uptake is aided by the increasing affinity of haemoglobin for oxygen, caused by falling P_{CO_2} and temperature and increased pH and reflected by a left shift of the curve. The P_{O_2} at which the haemoglobin is 50% saturated is known as the P_{50}. Under normal arterial conditions (pH = 7.4, P_{CO_2} = 5.3 kPa or 40 mmHg, temperature = 37°C) P_{50} = 3.5 kPa (26.3 mmHg); right

shifts raise the P_{50} and left shifts lower it. A rise in the concentration of **2,3-di(or bi)phosphoglycerate** (2,3-DPG), which is a by-product of glycolysis in red cells, also causes a right shift. A rise in 2,3-DPG occurs in anaemia, causing a modest increase in P_{50}. Blood bank storage causes progressive depletion of 2,3-DPG and an undesirable left shift, but this can be minimized by storing the blood with citrate-phosphate-dextrose.

Anaemia and carbon monoxide poisoning

In **anaemia**, at any given P_{O_2}, the oxygen content is reduced because of the reduced concentration of binding sites. Figure 8c shows the dissociation curve for normal blood and for blood with [Hb] = 7.5 g/dL. Alveolar and arterial P_{O_2} is normal in anaemia and therefore arterial O_2 content is 10 mL/dL. At rest, the tissues need to remove about 5 mL/dL from the blood passing through them. To achieve this mixed venous content, P_{O_2} will need to fall to about 5.3 kPa (40 mmHg) (A in Fig. 8c) when [Hb] = 15 g/dL and about 3.6 kPa (27 mmHg) (B) when [Hb] = 7.5 g/dL. The reduced venous and hence capillary P_{O_2} reduces the partial pressure gradient driving diffusion of oxygen to the tissues, which may become inadequate in exercise when oxygen consumption increases.

Figure 8c also shows the dissociation curve for blood that has 50% of oxygen-binding sites occupied by carbon monoxide (CO, dashed line). Arterial oxygen content is 10 mL/dL, but there is also an altered shape and leftward shift of the dissociation curve, because CO binding increases the affinity of the remaining (CO-free) sites for oxygen. This impairs oxygen release in the tissues. Mixed venous P_{O_2} will now have to fall to 2 kPa (15 mmHg) (point C) to release the 5 mL/dL required and this will greatly reduce the pressure gradient for diffusion. At about 50–60% **carboxyhaemoglobin**, symptoms of impaired cerebral oxygenation (headache, convulsions, coma and death) are severe, whereas anaemic patients with the same arterial oxygen content are typically asymptomatic at rest. Haemoglobin has a high affinity for CO (about 240 times that for oxygen), so breathing even low concentrations causes a progressive increase in the cherry-red carboxyhaemoglobin. A cherry-red complexion is sometimes a feature of CO poisoning, although pallor and **cyanosis** (discussed in Chapter 22) are more common.

Other respiratory pigments

Fetal haemoglobin, HbF, differs from **adult haemoglobin, HbA** in that there are two γ-chains instead of two β-chains. The HbF dissociation curve lies to the left of that for HbA, reflecting its higher O_2 affinity. This difference is enhanced by the **double Bohr shift**: in the placenta P_{CO_2} moves from the fetal to maternal blood, shifting the maternal curve further right and the fetal curve further left. The high affinity of HbF relative to HbA helps transfer oxygen from mother to fetus and even though blood returning from the placenta to the fetus in the umbilical vein has a P_{O_2} of only about 4 kPa (30 mmHg), its saturation is 70%. Oxygen transport in the fetus is also helped by a high [Hb] of about 170–180 g/L.

Myoglobin, the respiratory pigment found in muscle, is composed of a single haem group attached to a single globin chain. With no co-operative binding its dissociation curve is hyperbolic. It is also far to the left of HbA and its high affinity means that its oxygen store is only released when local P_{O_2} is severely reduced, for example in heavy exercise.

(a) CO_2 dissociation curve

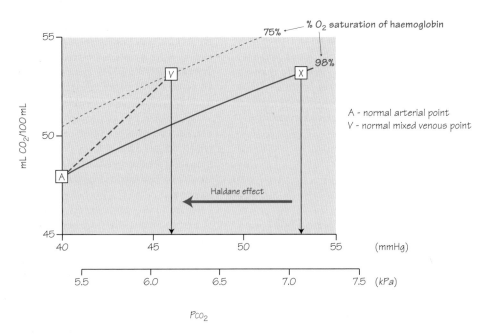

The solid line (A–X) shows what the relationship between blood P_{CO_2} and CO_2 content would be if Hb remained 98% saturated. However, as mixed venous blood Hb is only 75% saturated, more CO_2 can be carried for any given P_{CO_2} as shown by the dashed line A–V (the Halane effect; see text)

(b) CO_2 uptake and O_2 delivery in the tissues

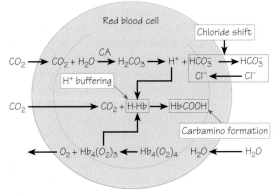

CA = Carbonic anhydrase

(c) Carriage of CO_2 in arterial and mixed venous blood

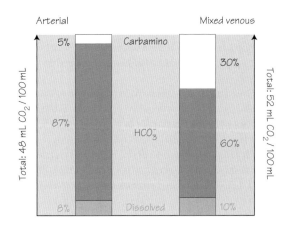

Carbon dioxide (CO_2) is produced by tissues and transported in the blood to the lungs, where it is expired. The amount of CO_2 that can be carried in the blood is much greater than that of O_2, as seen in the **CO_2 dissociation curve** (Fig. 9a). The CO_2 dissociation curve is also more linear and does not reach a plateau. CO_2 is transported in the blood as bicarbonate ions, as carbamino compounds combined with proteins or simply dissolved in the plasma (Fig. 9c).

Bicarbonate: In mixed venous blood about 60% of CO_2 is transported in the form of bicarbonate. CO_2 and water combine to form carbonic acid (H_2CO_3) and thence bicarbonate (HCO_3^-):

$$\overset{CA}{CO_2 + H_2O \Leftrightarrow H_2CO_3} \Leftrightarrow H^+ + HCO_3^- \tag{1}$$

The left-hand side of the equation proceeds slowly in plasma, but is accelerated dramatically by the enzyme **carbonic anhydrase** (CA), which is present in red blood cells. Ionization of carbonic acid to bicarbonate and H^+ is rapid in the absence of any enzyme. Bicarbonate is therefore formed preferentially in the red cells, from which it easily diffuses out into the plasma. The red cell membrane is, however, impermeable to H^+ ions and they remain within the cell. In order to maintain electrical neutrality, Cl^- ions diffuse into the cell to replace bicarbonate, an effect known as the **chloride shift** (Fig. 9b). A build-up of H^+ in the red blood cell would impair further movement of equation 1 to the right, thus limiting formation of bicarbonate. However, H^+ binds avidly to reduced (deoxygenated) haemoglobin, i.e. **haemoglobin acts as a buffer**, so the rise in H^+ concentration is limited and more bicarbonate can be formed. Oxygenated haemoglobin does not bind H^+ so well, as it is more acid. This contributes to the **Haldane effect**, which states that, for any given $P\text{CO}_2$, the CO_2 content of deoxygenated blood is greater than that of oxygenated blood. As a result, when blood gives up oxygen to respiring tissues, i.e. becomes deoxygenated, it is able to take up more of the CO_2 that the tissues are producing. Conversely, oxygenation of haemoglobin in the lung assists the unloading of CO_2 from the blood so it can be expired. This is illustrated by Fig. 9a and equation 2.

$$H^+ + haemoglobin \cdot O_2 \Leftrightarrow haemoglobin \cdot H + O_2 \tag{2}$$

Note that as a consequence of all the above, deoxygenated red cells have a higher intracellular osmolality and water enters, causing them to swell slightly. In the lung, CO_2 is given off, osmolality falls and the red cells shrink again.

Carbamino compounds: CO_2 combines rapidly with terminal amino groups on proteins to form carbamino compounds:

$$CO_2 + protein \cdot NH_2 \Leftrightarrow protein \cdot NH \cdot COOH \tag{3}$$

In blood, the most prevalent protein is haemoglobin, which combines with CO_2 to form carbaminohaemoglobin. Reduced haemoglobin forms carbamino compounds more readily than oxygenated haemoglobin and this also contributes to the Haldane effect (Fig. 9b). Around 30% of the CO_2 expired is carried to the lungs as carbamino compounds.

CO_2 in solution: CO_2 is ~20 times more soluble in water than O_2. A significant proportion (~10%) of the CO_2 exhaled is therefore carried to the lung dissolved in the plasma.

Because of the Haldane effect, the proportion of CO_2 that is carried in the blood as bicarbonate, carbamino compounds and simply dissolved differs between oxygenated arterial blood and deoxygenated mixed venous blood (Fig. 9c).

Hypoventilation and hyperventilation

Ventilation is normally closely matched to the metabolic requirements of the body and this can be estimated from the rate of CO_2 production (Chapter 11). The partial pressure of CO_2 in the alveoli ($P_A\text{CO}_2$) is proportional to the amount of CO_2 exhaled per minute ($V\text{CO}_2$) as a fraction of total alveolar ventilation (V_A), i.e. $P_A\text{CO}_2 \propto V\text{CO}_2/V_A$. The gas in the alveoli is in equilibrium with arterial blood, so $P_A\text{CO}_2$ estimates the partial pressure in the blood ($P_a\text{CO}_2$). At any given metabolic rate, doubling the alveolar ventilation halves alveolar and arterial $P\text{CO}_2$, and halving alveolar ventilation doubles $P_A\text{CO}_2$ and $P_a\text{CO}_2$. Changes in alveolar ventilation also affect alveolar $P\text{O}_2$, but the relationship is not as simple because O_2 is present in both inspired and expired gas. Thus doubling alveolar ventilation will halve the *difference* between the inspired and alveolar O_2 fraction. **Hypoventilation** (under-ventilation) and **hyperventilation** (over-ventilation) are therefore defined in terms of $P_a\text{CO}_2$, so that a patient is *hypoventilating* when $P_a\text{CO}_2$ >45 mmHg (5.9 kPa) and *hyperventilating* when the $P_a\text{CO}_2$ < 40 mmHg (5.3 kPa). Note that the CO_2 content of the blood will be affected more slowly by hypo- or hyperventilation than the O_2 content, as the CO_2 stores in the body (e.g. as HCO_3^-) are ~75 times greater than those for O_2 (e.g. haemoglobin, myoglobin). Also, although hyperventilation increases arterial $P\text{O}_2$, in a healthy patient it has little effect on O_2 content as arterial haemoglobin is normally close to saturation (Chapter 8).

Hypoventilation may occur when the respiratory drive is impaired by head injury, or drugs such as morphine or barbiturates which suppress the respiratory centres. It may also be caused by respiratory muscle weakness or severe chest trauma. Hypoventilation is sometimes a feature of severe chronic obstructive airways disease (COPD; Chapter 23), but is not usually a feature of asthma (Chapter 25) unless the attack is severe or prolonged enough to lead to exhaustion. Hypoventilation is difficult to achieve voluntarily, as the respiratory centres create an overwhelming desire to breathe. Hyperventilation can be induced voluntarily and in states of high anxiety or pain.

Hypoventilation leads to **hypercapnia** (high $P_a\text{CO}_2$) and **hypoxia** (low $P_a\text{O}_2$). Increasing severity of hypercapnia causes peripheral vasodilatation, muscle twitching and hand flap, confusion, drowsiness and eventually coma; there is a concomitant respiratory acidosis (Chapter 10). The effects of hypoxia are dealt with elsewhere (Chapter 8). A low $P_a\text{CO}_2$ as a result of hyperventilation causes light-headedness, visual disturbances due to cerebral vasoconstriction, paraesthesia ('pins and needles') and muscle cramps, especially carpopedal spasm.

Respiratory gas exchange ratio

Respiratory gas exchange ratio (R) is the ratio of CO_2 production to O_2 consumption as measured at the mouth. In the steady state, CO_2 production and O_2 consumption reflect tissue metabolism. Metabolizing carbohydrates produces a volume of CO_2 equal to the volume of O_2 consumed, whereas metabolizing fats and proteins produces a smaller volume of CO_2 than O_2 consumed. For an average mixed diet R ≈ 0.8.

(a) Relationship between P_{CO_2}, HCO_3^- and pH, and the Henderson–Hasselbalch equation

$$CO_2 + H_2O \Leftrightarrow H_2CO_3 \Leftrightarrow HCO_3^- + H^+$$

$$K = \frac{[HCO_3^-] \times [H^+]}{[H_2CO_3]} \quad \text{(From Law of Mass Action)}$$

⬇

$$\log K = \log [H^+] + \log \frac{[HCO_3^-]}{[H_2CO_3]}$$

K = dissociation constant;
K_A = corrected for $[CO_2]$ instead of $[H_2CO_3]$

⬇

$$-\log [H^+] = -\log K + \log \frac{[HCO_3^-]}{[H_2CO_3]}$$

Solubility (s) =
0.23 mmol / litre / kPa
0.03 mmol / litre / mmHg

⬇

$$pH = pK + \log \frac{[HCO_3^-]}{[H_2CO_3]}$$

⬇

But: $[H_2CO_3] \propto [CO_2]$ ($pK_A = 6.1$)
and: $[CO_2] = P_{CO_2} \times s$ (solubility)

⬇

$$pH = 6.1 + \log \frac{[HCO_3^-]}{P_{CO_2} \times s}$$

(b) Davenport diagram

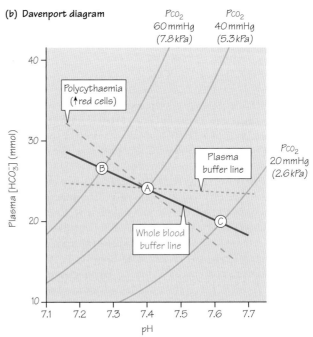

(c) Compensation and base excess

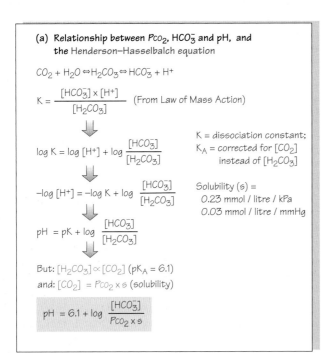

(d) Flenley acid–base nomogram

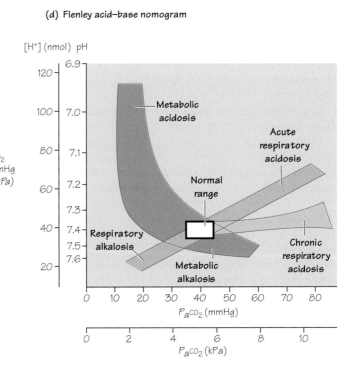

The pH of arterial blood is normally ~7.4 ([H$^+$] = 40 nmol). Regulation of **acid–base status** so that blood pH remains between 7.35 and 7.45 (45–35 nmol) is vital for the correct functioning of the body. Carriage of CO_2 in blood and its removal in the lungs (Chapter 9) has an important influence on acid–base status, as around 100 times more acid equivalents are expired per day in the form of CO_2/carbonic acid than are excreted as fixed acids by the kidneys. Nevertheless, renal mechanisms are important for regulation of acid–base balance, and for compensating respiratory disorders (see below).

Buffers bind or release H$^+$ according to the pH; this limits the change in pH that occurs when acid is added. The relationship between the amount of acid equivalent added to a solution containing a buffer and the resultant change in pH is known as the **buffer curve**. Buffers are most effective when pH is close to their pK$_A$ (log of dissociation constant, K$_A$; see Fig. 10a). The most important buffers in blood are **haemoglobin** and **bicarbonate** (HCO$_3^-$). CO_2 combines with water to form carbonic acid (H_2CO_3), which dissociates to HCO$_3^-$ and H$^+$ (Chapter 9). The relationship between pH, P_{CO_2} and [HCO$_3^-$] is described by the **Henderson–Hasselbalch equation** (Fig. 10a), where pK$_A$ is 6.1 and [CO_2] can be calculated as $P_{CO_2} \times CO_2$ solubility, which is 0.03 mmol·L·mmHg^{-1} (0.23 mmol·L·kPa^{-1}). In normal blood, [HCO$_3^-$] is 24 mmol and P_{CO_2} 40 mmHg (5.3 kPa) and pH calculates as 7.4. Whatever their actual values, the important points to remember are that if the ratio [HCO$_3^-$]/[CO_2] remains constant at 20, then pH will remain at 7.4, and:

$$pH \propto \log \frac{[HCO_3^-]}{P_{CO_2}}$$

Although the pK$_A$ of the bicarbonate system (6.1) is further away from blood pH (7.4) than would seem ideal for a buffer, the fact that P_{CO_2} and HCO$_3^-$ can be independently controlled by ventilation (Chapter 9) and the kidneys, respectively, means that in practice it makes an effective buffer system.

Haemoglobin is an important buffer, particularly when deoxygenated (Chapter 9) and significantly improves the buffering capacity of whole blood compared with plasma (Fig. 10b; the steeper the line, the better the buffering). All other **blood proteins** combined have <20% of the buffering capacity of haemoglobin.

Acidosis, alkalosis and compensation

The relationship between pH, HCO$_3^-$ and P_{CO_2} can be portrayed using a **Davenport diagram** (Fig. 10b). HCO$_3^-$ is plotted against pH for given values of P_{CO_2}. The line marked BAC is the **buffer line** for whole blood; in the absence of other changes (e.g. anaemia, polycythaemia), changes in P_{CO_2} alter HCO$_3^-$ and pH along this line. Point A represents normal conditions (pH 7.4, HCO$_3^-$ 24 mmol, P_{CO_2} 40 mmHg/5.3 kPa). An acute rise in P_{CO_2} (hypercapnia) due to hypoventilation (e.g. **acute respiratory failure**) will decrease the [HCO$_3^-$] : P_{CO_2} ratio and consequently pH (see above). This **respiratory acidosis** is represented by a move from A to B (Fig. 10c); A to C represents a **respiratory alkalosis** (e.g. hyperventilation). A sustained respiratory acidosis caused by **chronic respiratory failure** (Chapter 22) can be partially **compensated** by excretion of H$^+$ (as phosphate and ammonium) and reabsorption of HCO$_3^-$ in the kidneys. The [HCO$_3^-$] : P_{CO_2} ratio is thus largely

restored and pH returns towards normal. This **renal compensation** is described by the arrow between B and D (Fig. 10c). Conversely, a respiratory alkalosis may be compensated by increased renal excretion of HCO$_3^-$ (C to E).

The term **metabolic acidosis** (or **alkalosis**) is used when acid–base status is disturbed by changes in HCO$_3^-$ rather than CO_2—as a result, for example, of renal disease or increased H$^+$ production (Table). A **metabolic acidosis** (Fig. 10c, G) may be partially compensated by increased ventilation and a reduction in P_{CO_2} (G to E), initiated by detection of acid pH by the chemoreceptors (Chapter 11). There can be little **respiratory compensation** for **metabolic alkalosis** (F), as this may require unsustainable falls in ventilation.

Base excess

Measurement of pH alone gives little indication of acid–base status (Fig. 10d); although pH may be normal, P_{CO_2} and [HCO$_3^-$] may not be (D, E). Measurements of blood pH, P_{CO_2} and P_{O_2} are always taken clinically. **Base excess** or **base deficit** (negative base excess) is the millimole per litre of acid or alkali needed to titrate the blood back to a pH of 7.4. It is normally 0 ± 2 mmol/L. In a pure metabolic acidosis, it is greater than the difference between the actual and normal HCO$_3^-$, as haemoglobin and buffers must also be titrated. Base excess is normally calculated from the pH and P_{CO_2} automatically by clinical blood gas analysers, corrected for haemoglobin. The example in Fig. 10c is for a fully compensated respiratory acidosis (D) and gives an indication of the degree of renal compensation (i.e. after titration back to pH 7.4). Base excess may be useful for diagnosis, but should be used with caution as a basis for treatment, as the whole-body buffer line may differ significantly from that of blood *in vitro*, due to contributions from interstitial fluids (Fig. 10b).

Metabolic and respiratory acid–base disorders may often be combined, making diagnosis difficult. A common example is respiratory failure (Chapter 22), where concomitant hypoxia can cause metabolic acidosis in addition to the primary respiratory acidosis. A useful diagnostic aid is the **Flenley nomogram** (Fig. 10d). Only one type of disturbance is likely if the patient's arterial pH and P_{CO_2} fall within a band (95% confidence limits).

Common causes of acid–base disorders.	
Respiratory acidosis	Respiratory alkalosis
Airway obstruction	High levels of anxiety
Respiratory muscle disease	(hyperventilation)
Head trauma	Pain
	Altitude
	Excessive mechanical ventilation
Metabolic acidosis	Metabolic alkalosis
Loss of HCO$_3^-$ from gut (diarrhoea)	Volume depletion
Renal failure or tubular damage	Diuretics (loop, thiazide)
Lactic acidosis (hypoxia, sepsis)	K$^+$ deficiency
Ketoacidosis (diabetes, starvation)	Excess mineralocorticoids
	Vomiting, loss of stomach fluids

11 Control of breathing I: chemical mechanisms

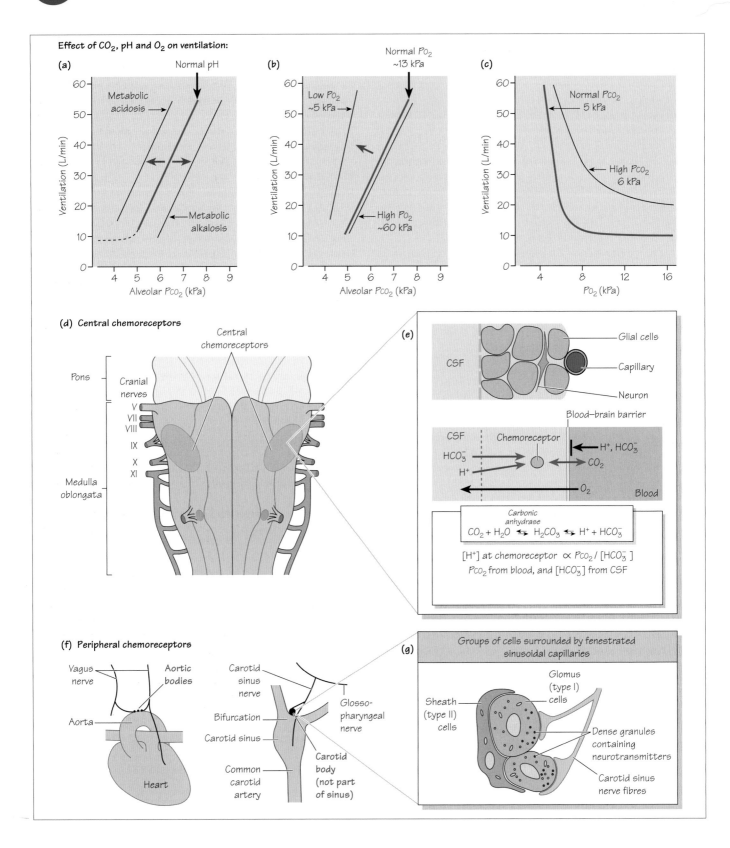

Effect of CO_2, pH and O_2 on ventilation:

(a) — Ventilation (L/min) vs Alveolar P_{CO_2} (kPa); Normal pH, Metabolic acidosis, Metabolic alkalosis

(b) — Ventilation (L/min) vs Alveolar P_{CO_2} (kPa); Normal P_{O_2} ~13 kPa, Low P_{O_2} ~5 kPa, High P_{O_2} ~60 kPa

(c) — Ventilation (L/min) vs P_{O_2} (kPa); Normal P_{CO_2} 5 kPa, High P_{CO_2} 6 kPa

(d) Central chemoreceptors

Central chemoreceptors
Pons
Cranial nerves
V
VII
VIII
IX
X
XI
Medulla oblongata

(e)
CSF — Glial cells, Capillary, Neuron
Blood–brain barrier
CSF — Chemoreceptor — H^+, HCO_3^-
HCO_3^- — CO_2
H^+ — O_2 — Blood

Carbonic anhydrase
$$CO_2 + H_2O \rightleftharpoons H_2CO_3 \rightleftharpoons H^+ + HCO_3^-$$

$[H^+]$ at chemoreceptor $\propto P_{CO_2} / [HCO_3^-]$
P_{CO_2} from blood, and $[HCO_3^-]$ from CSF

(f) Peripheral chemoreceptors

Vagus nerve
Aortic bodies
Aorta
Heart

Carotid sinus nerve
Bifurcation
Carotid sinus
Common carotid artery
Glosso-pharyngeal nerve
Carotid body (not part of sinus)

(g) Groups of cells surrounded by fenestrated sinusoidal capillaries

Glomus (type I) cells
Sheath (type II) cells
Dense granules containing neurotransmitters
Carotid sinus nerve fibres

Chemical control of ventilation is mediated via **central** and **peripheral chemoreceptors**, which detect arterial P_{CO_2} and pH (central and peripheral) and P_{O_2} (peripheral only), and modulate ventilation via a distributed network of neurones in the **brainstem** (Chapter 12). P_{CO_2} is the most important factor. The chemoreceptors allow arterial P_{CO_2} and P_{O_2} to be maintained within narrow limits despite large changes in metabolism (e.g. exercise).

Ventilatory response to changes in P_ACO_2 and P_AO_2

Normal alveolar P_{CO_2} (P_ACO_2) is ~5.3 kPa (40 mmHg). Increasing P_ACO_2 causes minute ventilation (litres ventilated per minute) to rise in an almost linear fashion (Fig. 12a), by ~15–25 L/min for each kPa rise in P_ACO_2 (~2.7 L/min/mmHg). There is considerable variation between individuals, and athletes and patients with chronic respiratory disease often have a reduced response to P_ACO_2 (Chapters 25 & 44). If P_ACO_2 increases above 10 kPa, ventilation decreases due to direct suppression of central respiratory neurones. A **metabolic acidosis** (an increase in [H+] caused by reduced [HCO$_3^-$]; see Chapter 10) shifts the CO_2–ventilation response curve to the left, whereas a **metabolic alkalosis** shifts it to the right (Fig. 12a). Note that a rise in [H+] caused by increased P_{CO_2} is called a **respiratory acidosis**. Increasing P_AO_2 from the normal value of ~13 kPa (~100 mmHg) has little effect on the CO_2–ventilation response curve, but if the P_AO_2 is reduced, the slope of the relationship becomes steeper and ventilation increases more for any given rise in P_ACO_2 (Fig. 12b). When the effect of P_ACO_2 is investigated independently (at constant P_ACO_2), there is little increase in ventilation until the P_AO_2 falls below ~8 kPa (~60 mmHg) (Fig. 12c). The effect of reducing P_AO_2 is, however, potentiated if the P_ACO_2 is raised—i.e. there is a **synergistic** (more than additive) relationship between the effects of P_AO_2 and P_ACO_2.

The central chemoreceptor

The **central chemoreceptor** consists of a diffuse collection of neurones located near the ventrolateral surface of the medulla, close to the exit of the ninth and tenth cranial nerves (Fig. 12d). These are sensitive to the pH of the surrounding cerebrospinal fluid (CSF) and do **not** respond to P_{O_2}. CSF is separated from blood by the **blood–brain barrier**, a tight endothelial layer lining the blood vessels of the brain. This barrier is impermeable to polar molecules such as H+ and HCO$_3^-$, but CO_2 can diffuse across it easily. The pH of CSF is therefore determined by the arterial P_{CO_2} and the CSF [HCO$_3^-$] (Chapter 10), and is not directly affected by changes in blood pH (Fig. 12e). CSF contains little protein, so its buffering capacity is low; therefore a small change in P_{CO_2} will cause a large change in pH. Stimulation of the central chemoreceptor by a fall in CSF pH (rise in blood P_{CO_2}) causes an increase in ventilation. The central chemoreceptor is responsible for ~80% of the response to CO_2 in humans. It has a relatively slow response time (~20 s), as CO_2 has to diffuse across the blood–brain barrier.

The peripheral chemoreceptors

The **peripheral chemoreceptors** are within the **carotid** and **aortic bodies**. The carotid body is a small (~2 mg) structure located at the bifurcation of the common carotid artery, just above the carotid sinus. It is innervated by the carotid sinus nerve, leading to the glossopharyngeal (Fig. 12f). The aortic bodies are distributed around the aortic arch and are innervated by the vagus. In humans, they are less important than carotid bodies. The carotid body contains **glomus** (type I) cells and **sheath** (type II) cells (Fig. 12g). Glomus cells are responsible for chemoreception; they have dense granules containing neurotransmitters and contact axons of the carotid sinus nerve. The function of sheath cells is unclear.

Carotid bodies respond to increased P_{CO_2} or [H+] and decreased P_{O_2} (**not** blood O_2 content) by increasing firing rate in the carotid sinus nerve, and thus ventilation. They have a high blood flow and consequently a small arteriovenous difference for P_{CO_2} and P_{O_2}. They respond rapidly (seconds) and are sufficiently fast to detect small oscillations in blood gases associated with breathing. The mechanisms by which changes in P_{CO_2}, pH and P_{O_2} are detected are unclear, but for P_{O_2} they are believed to involve inhibition of K+ channels in the glomus cell, with consequent depolarization, Ca^{2+} entry and release of neurotransmitters in the dense granules.

Adaptation: chronic respiratory disease and altitude

When hypercapnia (raised arterial P_{CO_2}) is prolonged, for example in chronic respiratory disease, CSF pH gradually returns to normal due to an adaptive increase in HCO$_3^-$ transport across the blood–brain barrier. The drive to breathe from the central chemoreceptor is consequently reduced, even though P_{CO_2} is still high. Associated with this, there is occasionally a loss of sensitivity to further increases in P_aCO_2, and the patient's ventilation is then primarily controlled by the level of P_{O_2} (**hypoxic drive**). Care must be taken with such patients, as giving high concentrations of O_2 in order to increase blood O_2 saturation may raise the P_{O_2} sufficiently to depress the hypoxic drive and hence ventilation. Normally, ~24–28% O_2 is given to such patients. This leads to a sufficiently small rise in P_aCO_2 as to have little effect on the hypoxic drive, but because of the steep slope of the O_2 dissociation curve (Chapter 8) it can result in a significant improvement in O_2 content. At high altitudes, ventilation is stimulated by the low atmospheric P_{O_2}. This leads to **hypocapnia** and alkalosis (as CO_2 is blown off), which depress ventilation. Over some days, the pH of CSF returns to normal due to HCO$_3^-$ transport out of the CSF, even though the P_{CO_2} remains low and ventilation increases again. Over a longer period, blood pH returns to normal due to renal compensation (Chapter 10). These processes form part of the **acclimatization to altitude**.

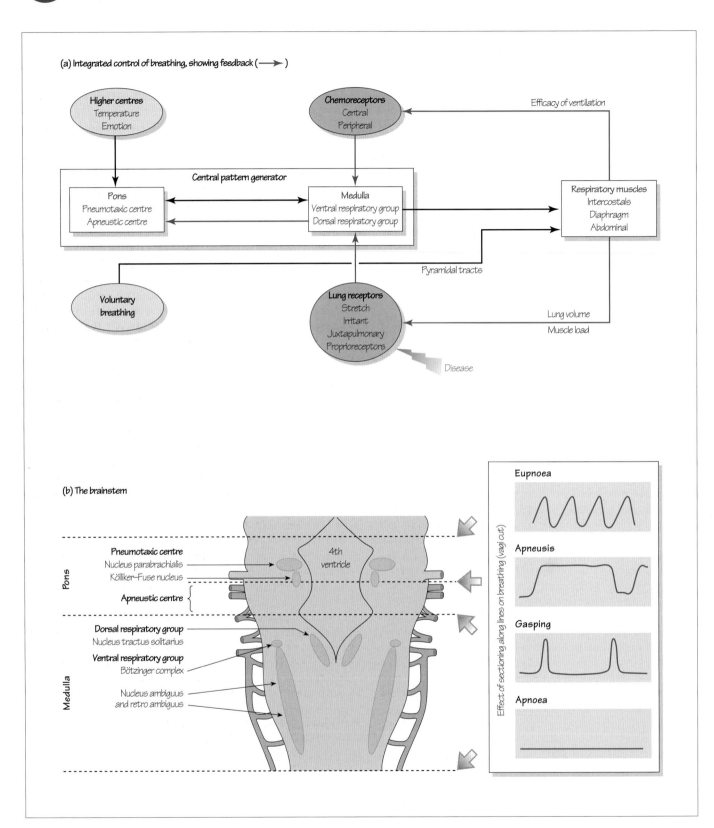

(a) Integrated control of breathing, showing feedback (⟶)

Higher centres
Temperature
Emotion

Chemoreceptors
Central
Peripheral

Efficacy of ventilation

Central pattern generator

Pons
Pneumotaxic centre
Apneustic centre

Medulla
Ventral respiratory group
Dorsal respiratory group

Respiratory muscles
Intercostals
Diaphragm
Abdominal

Pyramidal tracts

Voluntary
breathing

Lung receptors
Stretch
Irritant
Juxtapulmonary
Proprioreceptors

Lung volume
Muscle load

Disease

(b) The brainstem

Pons
Pneumotaxic centre
Nucleus parabrachialis
Kölliker–Fuse nucleus
Apneustic centre

4th ventricle

Medulla
Dorsal respiratory group
Nucleus tractus solitarius
Ventral respiratory group
Bötzinger complex
Nucleus ambiguus
and retro ambiguus

Effect of sectioning along lines on breathing (vagi cut)

Eupnoea

Apneusis

Gasping

Apnoea

Control of breathing involves a **central pattern generator** in the brainstem that sets the basic rhythm and pattern of ventilation and controls the respiratory muscles. It is modulated by higher centres and feedback from **sensors**, including **chemoreceptors** (Chapter 11) and lung **mechanoreceptors** (Fig. 12a). The neural networks involved are complex, reflecting the need to coordinate ventilation with functions such as coughing, swallowing and vocalization.

Brainstem and central pattern generator

The **central pattern generator** is a complex network encompassing diffuse groups of respiratory neurones in the pons and medulla. These groups contain **inspiratory** and **expiratory** neurones, with activity corresponding with inspiration and expiration, although others show more complex relationships. **Reciprocal inhibition** means that activity of inspiratory neurones inhibits activity in expiratory neurones, and vice versa.

The **medulla** contains two groups of respiratory neurones. The **dorsal respiratory group** (DRG) in the **nucleus tractus solitarii** contains inspiratory neurones and receives ascending input from central and peripheral chemoreceptors (Chapter 11), and from lung receptors via the vagus (Fig. 12a). The ventrolateral medulla contains a column of neurones extending from the lateral reticular nucleus and through the **nucleus ambiguus**, comprising the **caudal** (expiratory neurones) and **rostral** (inspiratory neurones) **ventral respiratory groups** (VRG) and **pre-Bötzinger** and **Bötzinger** complexes. Although the pre-Bötzinger complex contains neurones with intrinsic activity (pacemakers), these may only be associated with **gasping**, an autoresuscitative mechanism following hypoxia, as sectioning between the medulla and pons tends to abolish eupnoea (normal breathing) and lead to gasping in the absence of vagal input (Fig. 12b). Descending output from the medulla regulates activity of respiratory muscle motor neurones (intercostals, phrenic (diaphragm), abdominal).

The **pneumotaxic centre** is located in the **nucleus parabrachialis** and **Kölliker–Fuse nucleus** of the **pons**, and has a critical role in eupnoea and mediating responses to lung receptor stimulation (see below). It receives ascending input from the VRG, although vagal input from lung stretch receptors is routed via the DRG. The input from stretch receptors is important for timing of respiratory rhythm and especially switching inspiration off as lung volume increases. In the absence of vagal input sectioning the mid-pons leads to **apneusis** (prolonged inspiratory effort) (Fig. 12b), implying an **apneustic centre** in the caudal pons (*possibly associated with Kölliker–Fuse nucleus*). Descending input from the hypothalamus and higher centres mediates the effects of factors such as emotion and temperature on breathing, but eupnoea is maintained following sectioning above the pons (Fig. 12b), although voluntary control is lost. **Voluntary** control of breathing is mediated by motor neurones from the cortex contained in the **pyramidal tracts**, which bypass the pneumotaxic and medullary respiratory areas (Fig.12a). Certain rare brainstem lesions can leave the voluntary pathways intact while impairing brainstem mechanisms, so ventilation may cease when the patient falls asleep ('*Ondine's curse*'; Chapter 43).

The **origin of the respiratory rhythm** is controversial. Whereas some place this in the VRG and pre-Bötzinger complex, others suggest a '*switching concept*', with eupnoea reflecting the output of a pontomedullary neuronal circuit that includes pneumotaxic and apneustic centres, VRG and DRG. In either case, cycling or switching due to reciprocal inhibition and 'off switches' within these networks is probably the source of the rhythm of breathing rather than specific pacemaker neurones.

Lung receptors and reflexes

Stretch receptors: located in smooth muscle of the bronchial walls. These are mostly **slowly adapting** (continue to fire with sustained stimulation). Their afferent nerves ascend via the vagus. Stimulation of stretch receptors causes inspiration to be shorter and shallower and delays the next cycle. These receptors are largely responsible for the **Hering–Breuer inspiratory reflex**, where lung inflation inhibits inspiratory muscle activity. Conversely, the **deflation reflex** augments inspiratory muscle activity on lung deflation. These reflexes are weak during normal breathing in adults, but become more relevant when tidal volume is large (>1 L, e.g. in exercise). The reflex is very sensitive in neonates to protect the lungs against over-inflation due to the highly compliant nature of the chest wall.

Juxtapulmonary or 'J' receptors: located on alveolar and bronchial walls, close to the capillaries. Their afferents are small unmyelinated (C-fibre) or myelinated nerves in the vagus. Activation causes **apnoea** (cessation of breathing) or rapid shallow breathing, falls in heart rate and blood pressure, laryngeal constriction and relaxation of skeletal muscles. J receptors are stimulated by increased alveolar wall fluid, pulmonary congestion and oedema, microembolisms and inflammatory mediators such as histamine, all of which are associated with lung disease. The general action of J receptors is depression of somatic and visceral activity, which may be appropriate for serious lung damage as this would suppress metabolism in the face of compromised gas exchange.

Irritant receptors: located throughout airways between epithelial cells, with rapidly adapting afferent myelinated fibres in the vagus. Receptors in the trachea lead to cough; those in lower airways to hyperpnoea. They also cause reflex bronchial and laryngeal constrictions. Irritant receptors are stimulated by irritant gases, smoke and dust (Chapters 18 & 31), but also by rapid large inflations and deflations, airway deformation, pulmonary congestion and inflammation. Irritant receptors are responsible for the deep augmented breaths or sighs seen every 5–20 min at rest, which reverse the slow collapse of the lungs that occurs in quiet breathing. They may be involved with the first deep gasps of the newborn ('first breath') and the Hering–Breuer deflationary reflex.

Proprioceptors (position/length sensors): located in the Golgi tendon organs, muscle spindles and joints of the respiratory muscles. Afferents lead to the spinal cord via dorsal roots. Stimulated by shortening and load in respiratory muscles, although not diaphragm. They are important for coping with increased load and achieving optimal tidal volume and frequency. Input from non-respiratory muscles and joints can also stimulate breathing, for example during exercise.

Other receptors that may modulate respiration:

Pain receptors: stimulation often causes brief apnoea followed by increased breathing.

Receptors in the trigeminal region and larynx: stimulation may give rise to apnoea or laryngeal spasm.

Arterial baroreceptors: stimulation depresses breathing.

(a) Pulmonary and systemic circulation and normal anatomical right-to-left shunts

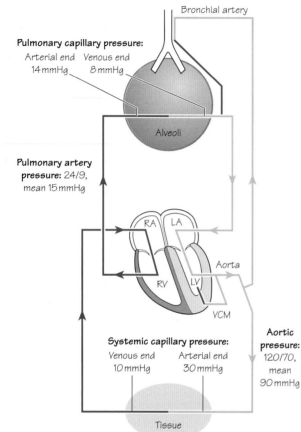

Bronchial artery

Pulmonary capillary pressure:
Arterial end 14 mmHg   Venous end 8 mmHg

Alveoli

Pulmonary artery pressure: 24/9, mean 15 mmHg

RA   LA

Aorta

RV   LV

VCM

Systemic capillary pressure:
Venous end 10 mmHg   Arterial end 30 mmHg

Aortic pressure: 120/70, mean 90 mmHg

Tissue

VCM = venae cordis minimae (Thebesian veins)

● ■ Normal O_2 and CO_2 pressures and contents

○ □ O_2 and CO_2 pressures and contents following mixing 20% mixed venous blood with 80% blood undergoing normal gas exchange

(b) The initial effects of a 20% right-to-left shunt on arterial O_2 and CO_2 contents and partial pressures

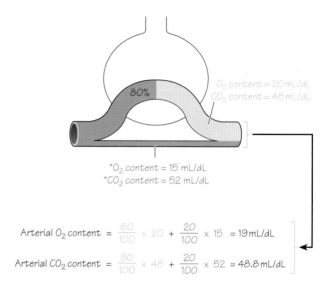

80%

O_2 content = 20 mL/dL
CO_2 content = 48 mL/dL

*O_2 content = 15 mL/dL
*CO_2 content = 52 mL/dL

$$\text{Arterial } O_2 \text{ content} = \frac{80}{100} \times 20 + \frac{20}{100} \times 15 = 19\,\text{mL/dL}$$

$$\text{Arterial } CO_2 \text{ content} = \frac{80}{100} \times 48 + \frac{20}{100} \times 52 = 48.8\,\text{mL/dL}$$

*Note: the mixed venous contents used are normal values. In fact the abnormal arterial contents would lead to abnormal mixed venous contents so this simple analysis underestimates the effects on arterial contents.

The Po_2 and Pco_2 that result from these O_2 and CO_2 contents can be found from the O_2 and CO_2 dissociation curves:

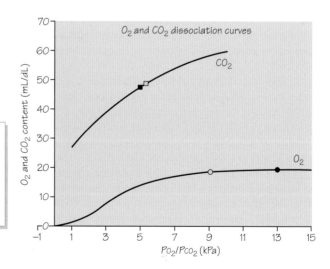

O_2 and CO_2 dissociation curves

CO_2

O_2

O_2 and CO_2 content (mL/dL)

Po_2/Pco_2 (kPa)

Pulmonary circulation compared with the systemic circulation (Fig. 13a)

The **pulmonary circulation** is in series with the **systemic circulation** and pulmonary blood flow nearly equals aortic blood flow. **Pulmonary vascular resistance** is only about one-sixth of systemic resistance and the thin-walled right ventricle need only generate a mean **pulmonary artery pressure** of about 15 mmHg to drive the cardiac output through the lungs. Systemic pressures are higher (Fig. 13a), dropping steeply across the main resistance vessel, the arteriole, to give a capillary flow which is usually non-pulsatile. Pulmonary vascular resistance is more evenly distributed in the microcirculation and pulmonary capillary flow remains pulsatile.

Local systemic resistance and blood flow are controlled by sympathetic nerves, metabolites and other substances acting on arterioles. Both sympathetic and parasympathetic nerves innervate pulmonary vessels, but their influence is weak in most circumstances. Systemic arterioles dilate in response to hypoxia, increasing flow and hence oxygen delivery. In contrast, **hypoxic vasoconstriction** occurs in the pulmonary circulation. This response, which is accentuated by high $P\text{CO}_2$, improves gas exchange by diverting blood from underventilated to well-ventilated regions (Chapter 14). The response is unhelpful in the presence of global lung hypoxia, at altitude or in respiratory failure, where it may contribute to the development of pulmonary hypertension and right heart failure.

As cardiac output increases in exercise, pulmonary vascular resistance falls, as vessels are recruited and distended and the rise in pulmonary arterial pressure is small. The pulmonary circulation acts as a blood reservoir and the volume it contains varies, being about 450 mL when upright and 800 mL when lying down. Inspiration also increases pulmonary vascular volume.

Fluid balance across capillaries is determined by hydrostatic and oncotic pressures (the **Starling forces**; see *The Cardiovascular System at a Glance*) across capillary walls. **Capillary oncotic pressure** opposes filtration and is about 27 mmHg in both circulations. Although hydrostatic pressure is low in the pulmonary capillaries (about 10 mmHg), net filtration of fluid occurs in pulmonary capillaries as it does in systemic capillaries. Other factors favouring filtration are **interstitial oncotic pressure**, which is relatively high in the lungs (about 18 mmHg) and **interstitial hydrostatic pressure**, which is negative (about −4 mmHg). **Pulmonary oedema** occurs when these forces are altered to increase net filtration above the rate that can be cleared by the pulmonary lymphatics. For example, it may occur when pulmonary capillary pressure is increased in **mitral stenosis** and **left ventricular failure**. **Inspiratory crepitations** (crackles) on auscultation in these conditions are probably caused by popping open of airways in lungs stiffened by congestion with blood. They are most obvious at the bases, where hydrostatic pressure is highest. Pulmonary congestion and oedema are worsened by the increase in pulmonary blood volume lying down.

Anatomical or true right-to-left shunts

Ideally, all venous blood emerging from tissues would return to the right side of the heart to be pumped through the gas-exchanging lung. In fact, part of the blood draining the **bronchial circulation** joins the pulmonary vein. This part results in deoxygenated blood from the airways contaminating blood returning from alveoli (Fig. 13a). In addition, a small amount of the coronary venous blood drains directly into the left ventricular cavity via the **venae cordis minimae (Thebesian veins)**. These additions of deoxygenated (right-sided) blood to oxygenated (left-sided) blood are known as anatomical **right-to-left shunts**. In normal people, they are equivalent to 2% or less of the cardiac output, but they explain why arterial $P\text{O}_2$ is less than alveolar $P\text{O}_2$ even though pulmonary capillary blood equilibrates with alveolar gas.

In disease, right-to-left shunting of blood may be much larger. **Atelectasis** (airless lung) or **consolidation** in **pneumonia** will result in pulmonary arterial blood supplying the affected region failing to undergo gas exchange. Right-to-left shunts are also the cause of reduced arterial oxygenation in **cyanotic congenital heart disease** such as **tetralogy of Fallot**. Atrial or ventricular septal defects do not usually cause impaired gas exchange and cyanosis, as the higher left-sided pressures give rise to **left-to-right shunts** in which some oxygenated blood is pumped again through the lungs.

Effect of right-to-left shunts on arterial blood gases

In the right-to-left shunt shown schematically in Fig. 13b, 20% of blood fails to pass through functioning alveoli and its O_2 and CO_2 contents remain at mixed venous levels of 15 and 52 mL/dL, respectively. Eighty per cent of the blood undergoes normal gas exchange, emerging with normal O_2 and CO_2 contents of 20 and 48 mL/dL, respectively. The initial effect on arterial gas contents is calculated from a weighted average of the contents in these two blood streams. This gives an arterial O_2 content 1 mL/dL below normal and CO_2 content 0.8 mL/dL above normal. From the flat part of the oxygen dissociation curve, it can be seen that the resulting arterial $P\text{O}_2$ is about 9 kPa (68 mmHg) compared with the normal 13 kPa (97 mmHg). The much steeper CO_2 dissociation curve means the rise in $P\text{CO}_2$ is small, from the normal value of 5.3 kPa (40 mmHg) to about 5.5 kPa (41 mmHg).

If the respiratory system is otherwise normal, the reduced $P_a\text{O}_2$ and increased $P_a\text{CO}_2$ simulate ventilation via the chemoreceptors and CO_2 washed out of the functioning areas restores arterial CO_2 content and $P_a\text{CO}_2$ to normal. In contrast, increased ventilation has little effect on arterial oxygen content and $P\text{O}_2$, as blood draining the ventilated areas of the lung was already saturated. If hypoxia is severe, the stimulation in ventilation is often great enough to reduce $P_a\text{CO}_2$ below normal. Typically, in a right-to-left shunt there is a low $P_a\text{O}_2$ with a normal or low $P_a\text{CO}_2$.

14 Ventilation–perfusion mismatching

(a) Different types of V_A/Q regions

Normal	Dead space	Dead space effect	Shunt effect	True/anatomical shunt
$\dot{V}_A$ = Normal	$\dot{V}_A$ = Normal	$\dot{V}_A$ = Normal	$\dot{V}_A$ = Low	$\dot{V}_A$ = 0
$\dot{Q}$ = Normal	$\dot{Q}$ = 0	$\dot{Q}$ = Low	$\dot{Q}$ = Normal	$\dot{Q}$ = Normal
V_A/Q = Normal (close to 1)	$V_A/Q = \infty$	V_A/Q = High	V_A/Q = Low	V_A/Q = 0

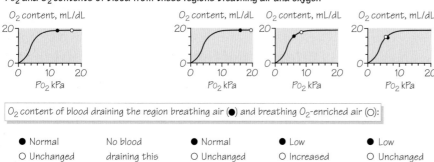

Po_2 and O_2 contents of blood from these regions breathing air and oxygen

O_2 content of blood draining the region breathing air (●) and breathing O_2-enriched air (○):

● Normal	No blood	● Normal	● Low	● Low
○ Unchanged	draining this region	○ Unchanged	○ Increased	○ Unchanged

(b) Variation of ventilation, $\dot{V}_A$, perfusion, $\dot{Q}$ and ventilation–perfusion ratio, V_A/Q with vertical height in the upright lung

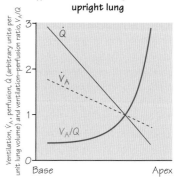

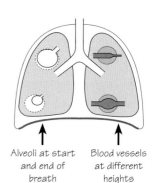

Alveoli at start and end of breath

Blood vessels at different heights

(c) The effect of a mixture of high and low V_A/Q regions on arterial blood gases

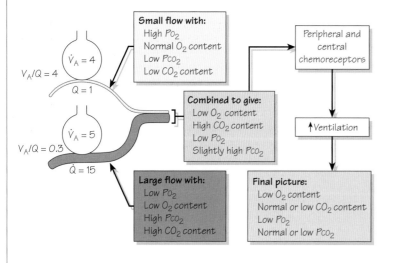

$V_A/Q = 4$

$\dot{V}_A = 4$

$\dot{Q} = 1$

Small flow with:
High Po_2
Normal O_2 content
Low Pco_2
Low CO_2 content

$V_A/Q = 0.3$

$\dot{V}_A = 5$

$\dot{Q} = 15$

Large flow with:
Low Po_2
Low O_2 content
High Pco_2
High CO_2 content

Combined to give:
Low O_2 content
High CO_2 content
Low Po_2
Slightly high Pco_2

Peripheral and central chemoreceptors

↑Ventilation

Final picture:
Low O_2 content
Normal or low CO_2 content
Low Po_2
Normal or low Pco_2

(d) Alveolar air equation

This predicts the Po_2 in the functioning or 'ideal' alveoli

$$P_AO_2 \cong P_{I}O_2 - \frac{P_aCO_2}{R}$$

R = The respiratory gas exchange ratio = $\dfrac{CO_2 \text{ production}}{O_2 \text{ consumption}}$

(R is usually about 0.8)

$P_{I}O_2$ = Inspired O_2 partial pressure
P_aCO_2 = Arterial CO_2 partial pressure (≈ alveolar)

At rest, alveolar ventilation and pulmonary blood flow are similar, each being around 5 L/min. Ventilation ($\dot{V}_A$) and perfusion ($\dot{Q}$) may vary in different lung regions, but for optimal gas exchange they must be matched. Areas with high perfusion need high ventilation and, ideally, local ventilation–perfusion ratios (V_A/Q) should be close to 1. Ventilation–perfusion mismatching or inequality is said to occur when regional V_A/Q ratios vary, with many being much greater or less than 1 (Fig. 14a). A right-to-left shunt from complete collapse or consolidation of a region (Chapter 13) has $V_A/Q = 0$, and can be viewed as an extreme example of ventilation–perfusion mismatching. At the other extreme, alveolar dead space from a pulmonary embolus is a ventilated region without perfusion and $V_A/Q = \infty$. Regions where V_A/Q is much greater than 1 have excessive ventilation or **dead space effect** and blood from them has a high P_{O_2} and a low P_{CO_2}. Regions with V_A/Q much less than 1 behave qualitatively like shunts and are sources of **shunt effect** or **venous admixture**. Blood draining them has undergone some gas exchange, but P_{O_2} is lower and P_{CO_2} higher than normal. The effect on P_{O_2} and O_2 content draining different V_A/Q regions both during air breathing and during oxygen breathing is shown in Fig. 14a (lower panel).

Effect of the upright posture on perfusion, ventilation and V_A/Q (Fig. 14b)

Hydrostatic pressure in all vessels varies with vertical height above or below the heart, because of the weight of blood. On standing, the increased pressure at the lung bases distends vessels, increasing flow. Pressures generated by the right heart are low and higher up the lung vascular pressures in diastole may fall below alveolar pressure at the venous end of the pulmonary capillary. In such regions, flow is reduced and determined by the difference between arterial and alveolar pressure. There may be regions at the apices—especially in haemorrhage or positive-pressure breathing—where alveolar pressure also exceeds pressure at the arterial end of the pulmonary capillaries. The vessels collapse completely for part of each cardiac cycle, giving low intermittent flow. The net result is a blood flow per unit volume of lung tissue that falls progressively from base to apex.

Gravity also affects intrapleural pressure, which is less negative at the base than the apex. As a result, at functional residual capacity apical alveoli are more expanded—with less capacity for further expansion during inspiration—than at the bases. Consequently, ventilation is also higher at the base than the apex. The effect of gravity on ventilation is less marked than on perfusion and so V_A/Q is higher at the apex than the base. In young people, this modest degree of mismatching has little effect on blood gases. The scatter of ventilation–perfusion ratios increases with age and contributes to the reduction in P_aO_2 seen in the elderly.

Ventilation–perfusion matching in disease

Increased ventilation–perfusion mismatching is an important cause of gas exchange problems in many respiratory diseases, including asthma, chronic obstructive pulmonary disease (COPD), pneumonia and pulmonary oedema. Regions of low V_A/Q may arise when airways are partly blocked by bronchoconstriction, inflammation or secretions and high V_A/Q in emphysematous areas where capillaries are lost. **Hypoxic vasoconstriction** (Chapter 13) helps reduce the severity of ventilation–perfusion mismatching.

Effect of ventilation–perfusion mismatching on arterial blood gases

Blood emerging from areas with high V_A/Q might be expected to compensate for blood from areas with low V_A/Q. This is not the case, for two reasons (Fig. 14c). First, although P_{O_2} will be increased in high V_A/Q regions, oxygen content is raised little, as blood is normally nearly saturated. Blood draining regions with low V_A/Q and low P_{O_2} (especially if <8 kPa, 60 mmHg) will have significantly reduced oxygen content. In addition, these areas contribute more blood than areas with high V_A/Q, which are typically caused by reduced perfusion. The net effect of mixing blood from areas with a wide range of ventilation–perfusion ratios is a low arterial O_2 content and P_aO_2. CO_2 content is less severely affected because the over-ventilated areas do lose extra CO_2 and partly compensate for low V_A/Q regions. Moreover, any abnormalities of P_aO_2 and P_aCO_2 will lead to a reflex increase in ventilation, which usually corrects or overcorrects the raised P_aCO_2 while being less effective at raising P_aO_2. The final arterial blood gas picture, a low P_aO_2 and a normal or low P_aCO_2, is similar to that resulting from anatomical right-to-left shunts (Chapter 13).

One difference is that arterial hypoxia caused by ventilation–perfusion mismatching improves much more with oxygen therapy than that caused by a shunt. In shunts, the **oxygen-enriched air** fails to reach the shunted blood. In V_A/Q mismatching, increased oxygen fraction can increase local P_{O_2} in areas of low V_A/Q (Fig. 14a), giving rise to significant improvement in arterial oxygen content and pressure.

Assessment of ventilation–perfusion mismatching

Regional ventilation and perfusion can be visualized by inhalation and infusion of appropriate radioisotopes (Chapter 21). A simple but useful index of the degree of mismatching is the difference between P_{O_2} in gas-exchanging or 'ideal' alveoli and in arterial blood. Ideal alveolar P_{O_2} can be calculated from the **alveolar air equation** (Fig. 14d). An increased **A–a P_{O_2} gradient** (A = alveolar P_{O_2}, a = arterial P_{O_2}) is usually caused by ventilation–perfusion mismatching or anatomical right-to-left shunts. In normal young people, there is a small A–a gradient (<2 kPa) arising from the normal anatomical right-to-left shunts discussed in Chapter 13.

Exercise, altitude and diving

Table 1
Typical values in healthy but sedentary 20-year-old man at rest and in max. exercise

	Rest	Maximal exercise
Heart rate (bpm)	70	200
Stroke volume (mL)	75	90
Cardiac output (mL/min)	5250	18,000
Arterial − mixed venous O_2 content* (mL/mL)	0.048	0.167
O_2 consumption (mL/min)	250	3000
Ventilation (mL/min)	7,500	140,000
Respiratory frequency (breaths/min)	15	56
Tidal volume (mL)	500	2,500

(*= O_2 extraction)

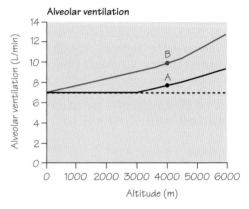

(b) Typical alveolar ventilation, Pco_2 and Po_2 at altitudes between sea level (0 m) and 6000 m for subjects exposed acutely (black solid line), and chronically (blue solid line) following acclimatization. The dashed line shows the values that would have occurred if alveolar ventilation remained at its sea level value.

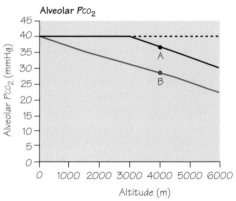

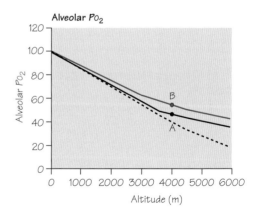

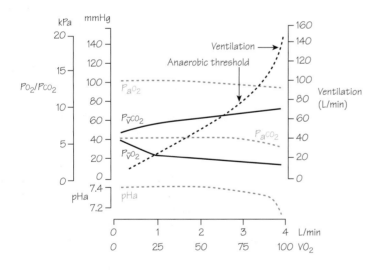

(a) Typical changes in ventilation, arterial Po_2 (P_aO_2), arterial Pco_2 (P_aco_2), arterial pH (pHa), mixed venous Po_2 (P_vO_2) and mixed venous Pco_2 (P_vco_2) in a fit young male as oxygen consumption is increased from its resting value of 0.25 L/min to his maximum oxygen consumption of 4 L/min.

Exercise

Resting arterial oxygen saturation is close to 100% and oxygen content cannot be raised significantly during exercise. **Oxygen delivery** (arterial oxygen content × blood flow) to exercising muscle is increased by increasing muscle blood flow, made possible by metabolic vasodilatation. **Oxygen extraction** from the delivered blood is also increased.

For the whole body, **oxygen consumption** (mL/min) = cardiac output (mL/min) × (arterial – mixed venous oxygen content) (mL/mL). In active muscle, oxygen unloading from haemoglobin is aided by the reduced tissue P_{O_2} and the rightward shift of the oxyhaemoglobin dissociation curve caused by local increases in P_{CO_2}, [H$^+$] and temperature. Maximum oxygen extraction does not vary greatly and the main factor determining **maximum oxygen consumption ($\dot{V}_{O_2}$ max)** is the maximum cardiac output. $\dot{V}_{O_2}$ max is an index of fitness and in a young man this might be 12 times resting oxygen consumption (Table 1) and more in an athlete.

In exercise, mixed venous blood has a reduced P_{O_2} and increased P_{CO_2}. As blood passes through the pulmonary capillaries, the increased alveolar to blood partial pressure gradients increase O_2 uptake and CO_2 output. In mild to moderate exercise, alveolar ventilation is accurately matched to metabolism and P_{aO_2}, P_{aCO_2} and arterial pH (pHa) are maintained at resting values (Fig. 15a). The mechanism(s) initiating and controlling the ventilatory response remain uncertain. In heavy exercise, increased anaerobic metabolism increases lactic acid production and reduces arterial pH. This gives an extra stimulus to breathing via the peripheral chemoreceptors and at this 'anaerobic threshold' the relationship between ventilation and oxygen consumption becomes steeper and P_{aCO_2} falls (Fig. 15a).

In some respiratory diseases, limited ability to increase ventilation or incomplete equilibrium in the pulmonary capillary may limit exercise.

Altitude

Barometric pressure falls progressively with increasing altitude from about 101 kPa (760 mmHg) at sea level to 33.6 kPa (252 mmHg) on the summit of Everest but oxygen fraction remains constant at 0.209. Moist inspired P_{O_2} ($0.209 \times (P_B - P_{H_2O})$) is about 19.9 kPa (149 mmHg) at sea level and about 5.7 kPa (43 mmHg) on Everest (Chapter 4).

If ventilation remains unchanged, reduced inspired P_{O_2} inevitably leads to reduced P_{aO_2} but P_{aCO_2} (α CO_2 production/alveolar ventilation) will be unaltered. This is the situation initially when a person ascends to altitudes up to about 3000 m (Fig. 15b). Hypoxic carotid body chemoreceptor stimulation occurs but any ventilatory increase lowers P_{aCO_2}, which depresses ventilation. Above 3000 m the more severe hypoxia does increase ventilation and P_{aCO_2} falls (Fig. 15b). **Acute mountain sickness** commonly develops some hours after rapid ascent to altitudes above 3600 m (12 000 ft) with symptoms such as fatigue, nausea, anorexia, dizziness, headaches and sleep disturbance. It can progress to life-threatening **high-altitude pulmonary oedema**

and/or **high-altitude cerebral oedema**, which usually require immediate descent. The more benign symptoms improve with time, a process known as **acclimatization**. Over the next few days, ventilation increases raising P_{aO_2} and lowering P_{aCO_2} (A to B, Fig. 15b). The initial alkalosis of arterial blood and cerebrospinal fluid (CSF) is corrected by bicarbonate transport out of the CSF and renal bicarbonate excretion. This reduces the inhibition of the central and peripheral chemoreceptors, allowing the ventilation to rise despite the low arterial P_{CO_2} and this lessens the hypoxia. **Erythropoietin** production by the kidney is stimulated by hypoxia and haemoglobin concentration rises from 150 g/L to around 200 g/L after a few weeks at altitude, aiding acclimatization by increasing arterial oxygen content.

At altitude the red blood cell **2,3 biphosphoglycerate** concentration increases and shifts the oxyhaemoglobin dissociation curve to the right. However, at very high altitude the very low P_{aCO_2} shifts the curve to the left and the beneficial effect of increased oxygen binding in the lungs seems to outweigh the impaired oxygen release in the tissues.

At altitude the widespread **hypoxia vasoconstriction** in the lungs is unhelpful. It increases pulmonary vascular resistance and those living at altitude may develop right ventricular strain and failure.

Diving

Diving into water affects the respiratory system in many ways. Breath-hold diving initiates several reflexes leading to the cardiovascular and respiratory effects of the **diving response**. Immersion of the face in water stimulates receptors around the eyes and nose supplied by the trigeminal nerves, leading to reflex apnoea, bradycardia and widespread vasoconstriction. The apnoea helps prevent water inhalation. The oxygen conserving bradycardia and vasoconstriction are enhanced by reflexes from the carotid body chemoreceptors but antagonized by reflexes from lung stretch receptors. The cardiovascular responses are usually modest in humans but excessive bradycardia sometimes occurs, especially following unexpected immersion during expiration and this may explain some accidental deaths in water.

The weight of the water increases the pressure on the body by 1 atmosphere (101 kPa, 760 mmHg) for every 10 m (33 ft) below the surface. Even 1 m below the surface breathing through a snorkel becomes difficult because the pressure on the chest opposes inspiration. In **SCUBA diving** greater depths are made possible by pressurizing the inspired, and hence alveolar gas, to ambient pressure but this brings other problems. Using compressed air the increased alveolar P_{N_2} raises arterial P_{N_2}, which has effects on the brain similar to alcohol intoxication and eventually leads to **nitrogen narcosis**. Dissolved nitrogen may also cause problems if the diver surfaces too rapidly. **Decompression sickness** or **'the bends'** occurs when the rapidly decreased pressure causes nitrogen to comes out of solution, forming bubbles in the blood and tissues, leading to musculoskeletal pains and neurological symptoms. If the diver fails to exhale while ascending the expanding gases can rupture the lungs.

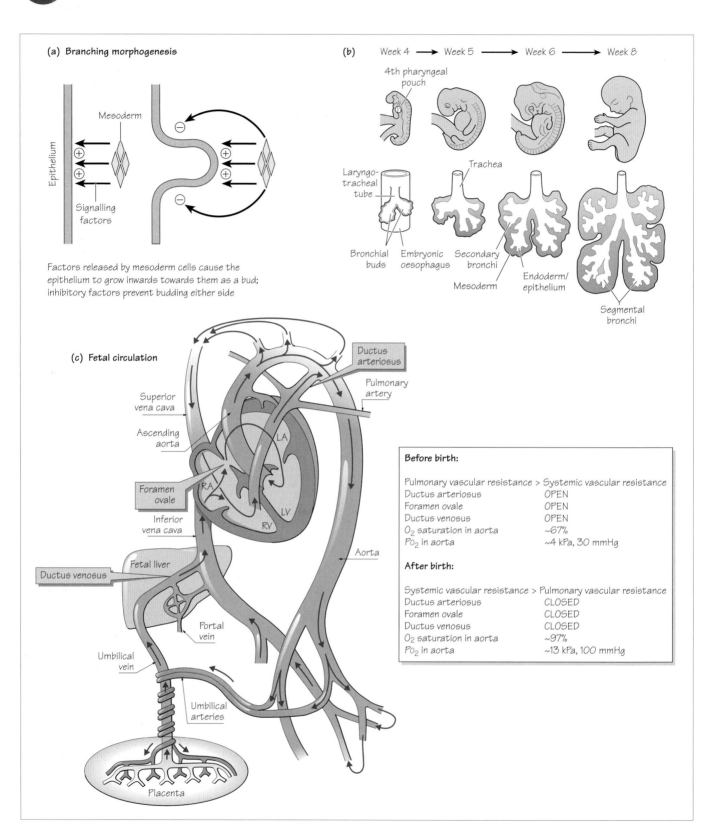

(a) Branching morphogenesis

Epithelium

Mesoderm

Signalling factors

Factors released by mesoderm cells cause the epithelium to grow inwards towards them as a bud; inhibitory factors prevent budding either side

(b) Week 4 ⟶ Week 5 ⟶ Week 6 ⟶ Week 8

4th pharyngeal pouch

Trachea

Laryngo-tracheal tube

Bronchial buds   Embryonic oesophagus   Secondary bronchi

Mesoderm   Endoderm/epithelium

Segmental bronchi

(c) Fetal circulation

Ductus arteriosus

Pulmonary artery

Superior vena cava

Ascending aorta

LA

Foramen ovale

RA

Inferior vena cava

LV

RV

Aorta

Fetal liver

Ductus venosus

Portal vein

Umbilical vein

Umbilical arteries

Placenta

Before birth:

Pulmonary vascular resistance > Systemic vascular resistance
Ductus arteriosus   OPEN
Foramen ovale   OPEN
Ductus venosus   OPEN
O_2 saturation in aorta   ~67%
Po_2 in aorta   ~4 kPa, 30 mmHg

After birth:

Systemic vascular resistance > Pulmonary vascular resistance
Ductus arteriosus   CLOSED
Foramen ovale   CLOSED
Ductus venosus   CLOSED
O_2 saturation in aorta   ~97%
Po_2 in aorta   ~13 kPa, 100 mmHg

The **embryological origins** of the lung are primitive **endoderm** of the foregut, which eventually forms the epithelium and glands of the larynx, trachea and lungs, and **splanchnic mesoderm**, which forms cartilage, smooth muscle, lung parenchyma and connective tissue. In common with many glandular organs, the lung develops by **branching morphogenesis** (Fig. 16a), with budding and branching of the endoderm/epithelium into mesoderm. The process requires reciprocal signalling between epithelium and mesoderm, with the mesoderm being primarily responsible for programming development of adjacent epithelium into the relevant structures. Many signalling molecules are vital for the orchestration of branching morphogenesis during lung development, including growth factors such as fibroblast growth factor (FGF), epidermal growth factor (EGF) and platelet-derived growth factor (PDGF); vascular endothelial growth factor (VEGF) is critical for pulmonary vascular development. Development of the respiratory system is generally divided into five stages or periods.

Embryonic period: the tracheobronchial tree originates from the **laryngotracheal tube**, below the fourth pharyngeal pouch at the caudal (tail) end of the primordial pharynx. The laryngotracheal tube starts to appear just prior to the fourth week of development, after the heart begins to beat. By the end of the fourth week, its end has bifurcated into two **bronchial buds**, progenitors of the two main bronchi and bronchial tree (Fig. 16b).

Pseudoglandular period (5th–17th weeks): the bronchial buds have now developed into the primordial left and (slightly larger) right primary bronchi, which subsequently divide by branching morphogenesis into five secondary bronchi (three right, two left). At the seventh week, these have started to branch progressively into 10 (right) or eight to nine (left) **segmental** (tertiary) bronchi, each of which eventually forms a **bronchopulmonary segment**. By the 17th week, most major structures of the lung have formed and are lined with columnar epithelial cells. Conducting blood vessels are present, but the gas-exchange surfaces have not yet developed and fetuses delivered during this period are therefore not viable.

Canalicular period (16th–25th weeks): bronchial cartilage, smooth muscle, pulmonary capillaries and connective tissue develop from the mesoderm. There is progressive differentiation and thinning of epithelial cells. The bronchi will have subdivided ~17 times after 24 weeks, finally forming the respiratory bronchioles which themselves divide into three to six alveolar ducts and some thin-walled **terminal sacs**. These are lined by very thin **type I alveolar pneumocytes** (squamous epithelium), which together with endothelial cells from capillaries form the future **alveolacapillary membrane** (gas-exchange surface). There are a few **type II alveolar pneumocytes**, secretory epithelial cells that produce surfactant. This reduces surface tension and allows expansion of the terminal sacs/alveoli (Chapter 6), but although it is present in small amounts from about the 20th week, there is insufficient to support unaided breathing until after 26 weeks (see **neonatal respiratory distress syndrome**, Chapter 17). Some gas exchange can occur at the end of this period, as there are both thin-walled terminal sacs and good vascularization, but the general level of immaturity means that fetuses born before the end of the 24th week normally die despite intensive care.

Saccular (terminal sac) period (24th week–parturition): associated with rapid development in the number of terminal sacs and the pulmonary and lymphatic capillary networks. Budding from terminal sacs and walls of terminal bronchioles and thinning of type I pneumocytes leads to formation of immature alveoli from around week 32. Sufficient surfactant and vascularization are normally present between the 24th and 26th week to allow survival of some premature fetuses, although this is very variable (Chapter 17). Surfactant increases significantly in the two weeks before birth.

Alveolar period (late fetal to childhood): clusters of immature alveoli form during the early part of this period; mature-type alveoli with thin interalveolar septa and gas-exchange surfaces do not appear until after birth. **Fetal breathing** movements are present before birth, with aspiration of amniotic fluid, and these stimulate lung growth and respiratory muscle conditioning. Lung development is impaired in the absence of fetal breathing, inadequate amniotic fluid (**oligohydramnios**) or space for lung growth (Chapter 17). The increase in lung size over the first 3 years is due primarily to an increase in number of alveoli and respiratory bronchioles; thereafter, both the number and size of alveoli increase. More than 90% of alveoli are formed after birth, reaching a maximum after 7–8 years. At the end of lung development, there are approximately 23 generations of airways, with ~17 million branches.

Fetal circulation and birth

Gas exchange in the fetus occurs in the **placenta**. Oxygen-rich blood from the umbilical vein flows into the liver and **ductus venosus**, and thus into the vena cava. Most blood entering the right atrium is diverted into the left atrium via the **foramen ovale**; the remainder enters the right ventricle and is pumped into the pulmonary artery as in the adult (Fig. 16c). However, the vascular resistance of the pulmonary circulation is high due to the collapsed state of the lungs and vasoconstriction, and 90% of the blood is therefore shunted via the **ductus arteriosus** into the aorta (Fig. 16c). Note that the P_aO_2 in the fetus is much lower (~4 kPa, 30 mmHg) than in the adult; oxygen transport is sustained by high-affinity fetal haemoglobin (Chapter 8).

At birth, the lungs are initially 50% full of fluid which is replaced by air. During and immediately following birth, fluid is removed via the pulmonary and lymphatic circulations, and through the mouth as a result of squeezing during delivery. Expansion and filling of the alveoli with air is critically dependent on the presence of **surfactant** to lower surface tension. The initiation of gas exchange in the lungs and consequent rise in blood PO_2 causes vasodilatation of the pulmonary circulation and constriction of the ductus arteriosus, so that blood from the right heart now follows its adult course via the lungs. The consequent fall in right atrial pressure causes the pressure gradient across the foramen ovale to reverse, causing functional closure within hours. The removal of venous return from the placenta also causes closure of the ductus venosus. Initially, pressure gradients keep the three fetal shunts closed, but after several months structural changes cause permanent closure. In 20% of adults this may remain incomplete for the foramen ovale, but is generally of no consequence.

Complications of development and congenital disease

(a) Relationship between prematurity and development of NRDS

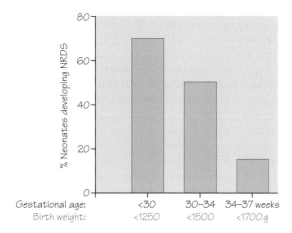

Gestational age: <30   30–34   34–37 weeks
Birth weight: <1250   <1500   <1700 g

Other factors such as socioeconomic status, maternal health, race and sex also affect incidence of NRDS

(d) Some genetic diseases in which the lung is a primary site of injury

Disease	Inheritance	Pathogenesis	Lung pathology
Alpha₁-antitrypsin deficiency	AD	Protease–antiprotease imbalance	Emphysema
Ciliary dyskinesia	AR	Impaired mucociliary clearance	Airway infection, bronchiectasis
Cystic fibrosis	AR	Abnormal chloride transport	Airway infection, bronchiectasis
Familial idiopathic fibrosis	AR	Unknown	Diffuse fibrosis
Lipoid proteinosis (Urbach–Wiethe syndrome)	AR	Lipoglycoprotein deposition in upper respiratory tract causing mucosal thickening and airway obstruction	Hyalinized or granular deposits in the tracheo-bronchial submucosa
Tracheobroncho-megaly (Mounier–Kuhn syndrome)	AR	Saccular bulges between cartilage rings resulting from atrophy of elastic and smooth muscle tissue and causing impaired mucociliary clearance	Recurrent airway infections
Congenital cartilage deficiency (Williams–Campbell syndrome)	?	Deficiency of subsegmental bronchial cartilage with airway collapse	Recurrent airway infections, bronchiectasis

AD = Autosomal dominant,   AR = Autosomal recessive

(b) Congenital diaphragmatic hernia

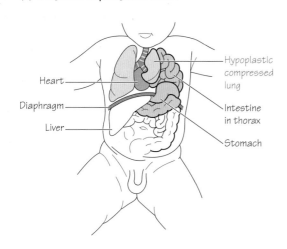

Heart
Diaphragm
Liver

Hypoplastic compressed lung
Intestine in thorax
Stomach

(c)

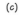
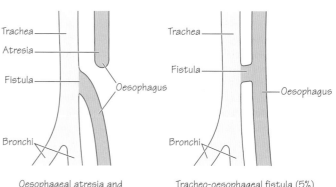

Trachea
Atresia
Fistula
Oesophagus
Bronchi

Oesophageal atresia and tracheo-oesophageal fistula (85%)

Trachea
Fistula
Oesophagus
Bronchi

Tracheo-oesophageal fistula (5%)

Problems associated with premature birth

Neonatal respiratory distress syndrome (NRDS), otherwise known as hyaline membrane disease, occurs in ~2% of all births and is characterized by rapid, laboured breathing and often sternal retraction due to partial collapse of the lungs after each breath. Lung compliance is low. NRDS is most commonly caused by lack of sufficient quantities of surfactant and consequent high surface tension in the alveoli and small airways. Incidence therefore increases sharply with degree of prematurity (Fig. 17a), although other factors may also reduce production of surfactant. When a premature birth is anticipated, the expectant mother can be treated with **corticosteroids** (betamethasone) to speed fetal lung development and surfactant production. Treatment with **exogenous surfactant** in the first 30 min after birth, either of natural origin or artificial, has also proved to be beneficial. Survival of neonates with NRDS often requires high positive-pressure mechanical ventilation and high levels of oxygen.

The large majority of NRDS cases are related to prematurity, with some due to other causes including damage to type II pneumocytes. A very few cases are due to a congenital absence of **pulmonary surfactant protein B**. These patients do not respond to any form of therapy and tend to die in the first few months of life.

Bronchopulmonary dysplasia (chronic lung disease of the newborn) is a long-term consequence of NRDS, primarily as a result of treatment with high positive-pressure ventilation combined with high levels of oxygen (hyperoxia). The condition is characterized by alterations in the structure and function of airways and pulmonary blood vessels, including increases in airway and vascular smooth muscle and obliteration of some microstructures. This leads to poorly reversible airway obstruction and sometimes pulmonary hypertension (high pulmonary blood pressure). Survivors may retain symptoms for many years, if not for life. There are several similarities to chronic obstructive pulmonary disease (COPD, Chapter 25) and chronic severe asthma in adults.

Several techniques have recently been designed to minimize the incidence of bronchopulmonary dysplasia in infants with NRDS. These include extracorporeal membrane oxygenation (**ECMO**), where blood is circulated via external apparatus for gas exchange; mechanical ventilation and hyperoxia are therefore not required and some success has been reported. Conversely, ECMO has not been found useful in adults with acute respiratory distress syndrome (ARDS, Chapter 40). **Partial fluid ventilation**, where the lungs are ventilated with fluids containing oxygen-carrying perfluorocarbons, has also been reported to be beneficial. Fluid ventilation circumvents problems associated with high surface tension by removing the air–liquid interface and allows small airways to open and contribute to gas exchange.

Congenital diseases

Congenital diaphragmatic hernia is the most common cause of lung hypoplasia (inadequate development of the lung), with an incidence of about one in 2000 births. Failure of the diaphragm to fuse with the membranes on the thoracic and peritoneal wall leads to a posterolateral defect, most commonly occurring on the left side (~85%), through which the abdominal viscera pass (herniate) into the thorax (Fig. 17b). This often includes the stomach, spleen and much of the intestines. The presence of the resultant mass severely restricts lung development and later inflation, leading to a significantly reduced lung volume and life-threatening breathing difficulties. The latter are the prime cause of death in congenital diaphragmatic hernia and most infants will die because the lungs are insufficiently developed to support life outside the uterus. Although surgical correction of the defect is possible both before and after birth, the mortality rate is very high. A related but very much less common condition is **eventration of the diaphragm**, where half the diaphragm lacks adequate muscle and bulges (eventrates) into the thoracic cavity. The viscera are forced into the pocket so formed, again restricting lung development.

Tracheo-oesophageal fistula (an opening between oesophagus and trachea) is the most common abnormality of the lower respiratory tract itself, with an incidence of about one in 4000 births. Its origins are located in the fourth week of development, when the embryonic respiratory tract starts to develop and divide from the embryonic oesophagus (Chapter 16). Eighty-five per cent of cases are associated with the descending part of the oesophagus having a blind ending (**oesophageal atresia**) (Fig. 17c); the lower part of the oesophagus joins instead to the base of the trachea. As a result, normal feeding is impossible and the gut becomes distended with air. There are also consequences *in utero*, as normally amniotic fluid is ingested by the fetus. Thus, oesophageal atresia is commonly associated with excess amniotic fluid (**polyhydramnios**), which can lead to severe defects in the central nervous system. Some 5% of cases of tracheo-oesophageal fistula show no atresia but only a fistula, and the remainder less common variations. Rare defects involving blockage or narrowing of the trachea itself (**tracheal atresia/stenosis**) are nearly always accompanied by various types of tracheo-oesophageal fistula.

There are many **inherited disorders of haemoglobin synthesis**. In some (e.g. **thalassaemia**) there is inadequate production of the normal globin chains and in others (e.g. HbS in **sickle cell disease**) there is production of globin chains with an abnormal amino acid sequence. They produce a variety of clinical problems mostly related to anaemia and/or alteration in the solubility (HbS) or oxygen affinity of the abnormal haemoglobin (Chapter 8).

Congenital influences on respiratory disease: several important respiratory diseases that are discussed in detail in other chapters have definite or implied genetic components, including asthma (Chapter 23), chronic obstructive pulmonary disease (Chapter 25), emphysema (Chapter 25), cystic fibrosis (Chapter 32) and primary pulmonary hypertension (Chapter 26). Other genetically linked diseases that cause pathological problems primarily in the lung are listed in Fig. 17d.

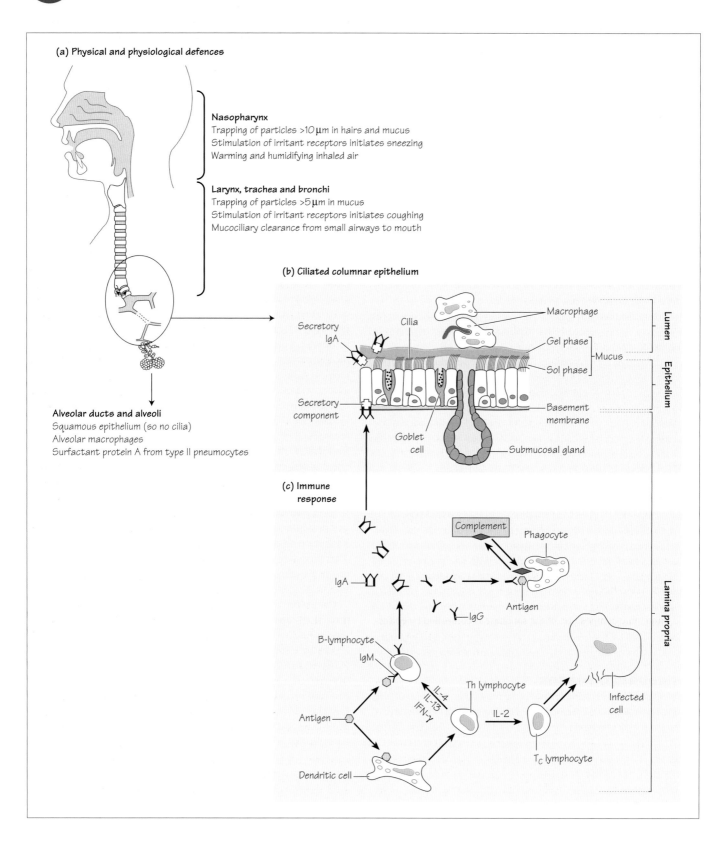

(a) Physical and physiological defences

Nasopharynx
Trapping of particles >10 μm in hairs and mucus
Stimulation of irritant receptors initiates sneezing
Warming and humidifying inhaled air

Larynx, trachea and bronchi
Trapping of particles >5 μm in mucus
Stimulation of irritant receptors initiates coughing
Mucociliary clearance from small airways to mouth

(b) Ciliated columnar epithelium

Secretory
IgA

Cilia

Macrophage

Gel phase

Sol phase

Mucus

Lumen

Epithelium

Secretory
component

Basement
membrane

Goblet
cell

Submucosal gland

Alveolar ducts and alveoli
Squamous epithelium (so no cilia)
Alveolar macrophages
Surfactant protein A from type II pneumocytes

**(c) Immune
response**

Complement

Phagocyte

IgA

Antigen

IgG

B-lymphocyte

IgM

Th lymphocyte

IL-4
IL-13
IFN-γ

IL-2

Infected
cell

Antigen

Lamina propria

T_C lymphocyte

Dendritic cell

Inhalation of air also allows ingress of dust, irritant particles and pathogens. The huge surface area of the lungs provides multiple opportunities for damage, and the warm humid environment provides ideal conditions for bacterial and other infestations. The respiratory tract, however, has a range of powerful defence mechanisms. Dysfunction of these mechanisms underlies many respiratory diseases, for example asthma (Chapter 23) and fibrosis (Chapters 29 & 31).

Physical and physiological defences

The nostrils and nasopharynx provide a physical barrier to particles >10 μm, in the form of hairs and mucus to which particles adhere (Fig. 18a). **Mucociliary transport** (see below) subsequently transfers these to the pharynx, where they are ingested. Only particles less than 5 μm generally get further than the trachea. The nasopharynx also provides important **humidifying** and **warming** functions for inhaled air, preventing drying of epithelium. Irritant particles in the nose and trachea, whether inhaled or transported from distal regions by mucociliary transport, stimulate irritant receptors (Chapter 12), provoking sneezing and coughing which eject foreign matter.

Mucus and airway secretions

The respiratory epithelium is covered with a 5–10 μm layer of gelatinous mucus (gel phase) floating on a slightly thinner fluid layer (sol phase) (Fig. 18b). The **cilia** on epithelial cells beat synchronously, and as they do so their tips catch in the gel phase and cause it to move towards the mouth, transporting particles and cellular debris with it (**mucociliary transport** or clearance). It takes ~40 min for mucus from large bronchi to reach the pharynx and from respiratory bronchioles several days. Many factors can disrupt this mechanism, including an increase in mucus viscosity or thickness, making it harder to move (e.g. inflammation, asthma), changes in the sol phase that inhibit cilia movement or prevent attachment to the gel phase and defects in cilia activity (**cilia dyskinesia**). Mucociliary transport is reduced by smoking, pollutants, anaesthetics and infection, and in **cystic fibrosis** (Chapter 32) and the rare congenital immotile cilia syndrome. Reduced mucociliary transport causes recurrent respiratory infections that progressively damage the lungs—for example, **bronchiectasis**, where the bronchial walls are thickened, permanently dilated and inflamed (Chapters 32 & 44).

Mucus is produced by **goblet cells** in the epithelium and **submucosal glands** (Fig. 18b). The major constituents are carbohydrate-rich glycoproteins called mucins which give mucus its gel-like nature. The fluidity and ionic composition of the sol phase is controlled by epithelial cells. Mucus contains several factors produced by epithelial and other cells or derived from plasma: **anti-proteases** such as α_1-**antitrypsin** inhibit the action of proteases released from bacteria and neutrophils which degrade proteins, and α_1-**antitrypsin deficiency** predisposes to disruption of elastin and development of emphysema (Chapter 25). **Surfactant protein A**, apart from its actions on surface tension, enhances phagocytosis by coating or **opsonizing** (literally 'making ready to eat') bacteria and other particles. **Lysozyme** is secreted in large quantities in the airways and has antifungal and bactericidal properties; together with the antimicrobial proteins lactoferrin, peroxidases and neutrophil-derived defensins, it provides non-specific immunity to the respiratory tract. **Secretory immunoglobulin A** (IgA) is the principal immunoglobulin in airway secretions and with IgM and IgG agglutinates and opsonizes antigenic particles; it also restricts adherence of microbes to the mucosa. Secretory IgA consists of a dimer of two IgA molecules produced by **plasma cells** (activated B lymphocytes, see below) and a glycoprotein **secretory component**. The latter is produced on the basolateral surface of epithelial cells, where it binds the IgA dimer (see Fig. 18b). The secretory IgA complex is then transferred to the luminal surface of the epithelial cell and released into the bronchial fluid (see Fig. 18b). It can account for 10% of the total protein in bronchoalveolar lavage fluid.

Lung macrophages

Macrophages are mobile **mononuclear phagocytes** that are found throughout the respiratory tract. They act as sentinels in the airways, providing innate protection against inhaled microorganisms and other particles by **phagocytosis** (ingesting them) and production of potent antimicrobial agents including reactive oxygen species. Phagocytosed organic material is usually digested, whereas inorganic material is sequestered inside the cell. As alveolar epithelium does not have cilia, alveolar macrophages are key to removing material and are the major cell present in the alveoli. Other functions include clearance of surfactant proteins and suppression of unnecessary immune responses by production of **anti-inflammatory cytokines** such as interleukin-10 (IL-10) and transforming growth factor β (TGFβ). However, in more severe infections, they can initiate inflammatory responses and by release of chemoattractants such as leukotriene B$_4$ promote neutrophil infiltration from the plasma. They can also act as antigen-presenting cells (see below).

Development of immunity

T and **B lymphocytes** migrate to lymph nodes, tonsils and adenoids and diffuse patches of bronchus-associated lymphoid tissue (**BALT**) within the lamina propria. Here they interact and are programmed. Antigen is presented to **CD4+ T lymphocytes** (T helper or T$_H$ cells) by **antigen-presenting cells**. The most important are **dendritic cells**, highly specialized mononuclear phagocytes (Fig. 18c). Macrophages, B lymphocytes and some epithelial cells can also act as antigen-presenting cells. On presentation of antigen, T$_H$ cells release **cytokines** such as IL-2, IL-4, IL-13 and interferon-γ (IFN-γ). IL-2 activates **CD8+ T lymphocytes** (cytotoxic or T$_C$ cells), which kill infected cells. IL-4, IL-13 and IFN-γ activate B lymphocytes in the presence of antigen binding to surface immunoglobulins (IgM) (Fig. 18). Activated B lymphocytes proliferate and differentiate into **plasma cells** that re-enter the blood stream. These secrete large amounts of antigen-specific antibody (immunoglobins). Binding of antibody to antigen may neutralize some toxic molecules, but more commonly activates secondary mechanisms, either directly by opsonization, allowing recognition and phagocytosis by macrophages and neutrophils, or by activation of **complement**. When activated, complement can: kill pathogens by lysis (bursting the cell membrane); opsonize the antibody–antigen complex; and recruit inflammatory cells. For more detailed information on immunity, see *Immunology at a Glance*.

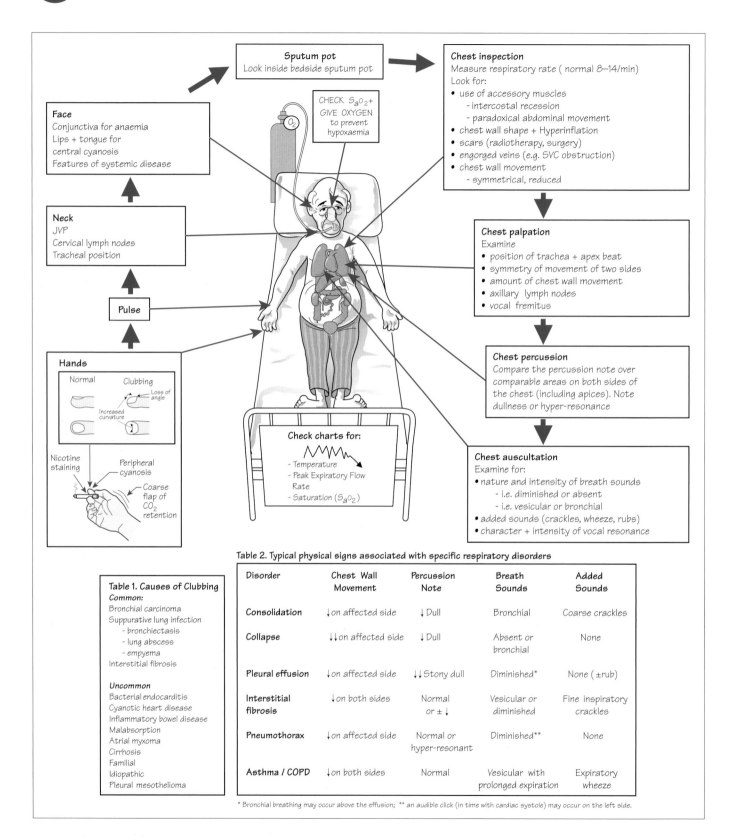

Sputm pot
Look inside bedside sputum pot

Chest inspection
Measure respiratory rate (normal 8–14/min)
Look for:
- use of accessory muscles
  - intercostal recession
  - paradoxical abdominal movement
- chest wall shape + Hyperinflation
- scars (radiotherapy, surgery)
- engorged veins (e.g. SVC obstruction)
- chest wall movement
  - symmetrical, reduced

CHECK S_aO_2+
GIVE OXYGEN
to prevent
hypoxaemia

Face
Conjunctiva for anaemia
Lips + tongue for
central cyanosis
Features of systemic disease

Neck
JVP
Cervical lymph nodes
Tracheal position

Chest palpation
Examine
- position of trachea + apex beat
- symmetry of movement of two sides
- amount of chest wall movement
- axillary lymph nodes
- vocal fremitus

Pulse

Hands

Normal   Clubbing
Loss of angle
Increased curvature

Nicotine staining   Peripheral cyanosis
Coarse flap of CO_2 retention

Chest percussion
Compare the percussion note over
comparable areas on both sides of
the chest (including apices). Note
dullness or hyper-resonance

Check charts for:
- Temperature
- Peak Expiratory Flow Rate
- Saturation (S_aO_2)

Chest auscultation
Examine for:
- nature and intensity of breath sounds
  - i.e. diminished or absent
  - i.e. vesicular or bronchial
- added sounds (crackles, wheeze, rubs)
- character + intensity of vocal resonance

Table 1. Causes of Clubbing
Common:
Bronchial carcinoma
Suppurative lung infection
- bronchiectasis
- lung abscess
- empyema
Interstitial fibrosis

Uncommon
Bacterial endocarditis
Cyanotic heart disease
Inflammatory bowel disease
Malabsorption
Atrial myxoma
Cirrhosis
Familial
Idiopathic
Pleural mesothelioma

Table 2. Typical physical signs associated with specific respiratory disorders

Disorder	Chest Wall Movement	Percussion Note	Breath Sounds	Added Sounds
Consolidation	↓on affected side	↓ Dull	Bronchial	Coarse crackles
Collapse	↓↓on affected side	↓ Dull	Absent or bronchial	None
Pleural effusion	↓on affected side	↓↓ Stony dull	Diminished*	None (±rub)
Interstitial fibrosis	↓on both sides	Normal or ± ↓	Vesicular or diminished	Fine inspiratory crackles
Pneumothorax	↓on affected side	Normal or hyper-resonant	Diminished**	None
Asthma / COPD	↓on both sides	Normal	Vesicular with prolonged expiration	Expiratory wheeze

* Bronchial breathing may occur above the effusion; ** an audible click (in time with cardiac systole) may occur on the left side.

History

A comprehensive history exploring the time-course, nature and severity of symptoms is the most important factor in establishing the cause of respiratory (or any other) disease. A systematic logical approach is outlined below and ensures a thorough, complete enquiry.

1 General features: age, sex, race and marital status are recorded as these may be associated with specific diseases. Thus, tuberculosis (TB) is more common in Asians, sarcoidosis in Afro-Caribbeans.

2 Presenting complaint: lists the main symptoms, usually chest pain, breathlessness, cough or haemoptysis in respiratory disease.

3 History of the presenting complaint: explores the specific features (e.g. onset, progress) of the main symptoms and associated systemic manifestations (e.g. fever, rigors, night sweats, malaise, weight loss, lymphadenopathy, arthritis, rashes). Thus, drenching night sweats and weight loss are associated with TB and cancer and erythema nodosum (inflammatory skin nodules) with sarcoidosis or TB. Obstructive sleep apnoea causes daytime sleepiness and is associated with snoring, obesity and collar size >17 inches (43 cm).

- *Chest pain:* establish site, sort (pleuritic, aching), severity, onset (gradual, sudden), periodicity (intermittent, constant), duration (minutes, days), aggravating and relieving factors (i.e. worse/better with breathing, posture) and time off work. Pleuritic pain is a localized, sharp pain aggravated by deep breathing.
- *Breathlessness:* occurs at rest, on exercise or when lying flat (orthopnoea). Determine rate of onset (sudden, gradual), when it occurs (i.e. nocturnal), exercise tolerance (i.e. when walking, running or climbing stairs?) and associated symptoms (e.g. hayfever, wheeze, stridor). In COPD breathlessness is worse on exercise. In contrast, breathlessness due to pulmonary oedema may suddenly wake a sleeping (i.e. supine) patient with heart failure. Nocturnal breathlessness with wheeze or seasonal breathlessness with hayfever suggest asthma.
- *Cough:* in the morning indicates chronic bronchitis (smoker's cough), at night suggests asthma or may be persistent after viral respiratory tract infections with bronchial hyper-responsiveness. Cough may be dry or productive of sputum. In a smoker, persistent cough, change in character or a bovine cough (due to recurrent laryngeal nerve palsy) indicates development of bronchial carcinoma.
- *Sputum:* morning cough and sputum production for 3 months a year for more than 1 year defines chronic bronchitis. Yellow or green, mucopurulent sputum occurs in chest infections and when copious and foul smelling may indicate bronchiectasis. Pink frothy sputum is typical of pulmonary oedema.
- *Haemoptysis:* determine frequency and quantity (i.e. flecks in sputum, fresh red blood); >500 mL haemoptysis in 24 hours is life-threatening. Infection (e.g. TB, pneumonia, bronchiectasis, *Aspergillus*) accounts for ~80% of haemoptysis; bronchial carcinoma and rarer causes (pulmonary infarction, vasculitis) for ~20%.

4 Past medical history: enquire about previous respiratory conditions; childhood whooping cough is associated with adult bronchiectasis; TB may reactivate in later life. Atopy and eczema are often associated with asthma. Assess understanding of current diseases and compliance with medications. Review previous chest X-rays, hospital admissions and the need for mechanical ventilation.

5 Medications: review current and previous medications, including inhalers, nebulizers and oxygen. Determine whether recent changes are associated with new symptoms (e.g. β-blockers may precipitate or worsen asthma; cytotoxics (e.g. methotrexate) can cause pulmonary fibrosis). Record **allergies** to medications and foods.

6 Family, occupational and social history: a family history of atopy, tuberculosis, COPD or cystic fibrosis may help establish a diagnosis. **Smoking history** including duration and amount (1 pack/day for 1 year = 1 pack/year). **Alcohol abuse** predisposes to tuberculosis. **Occupation** may predispose to respiratory disease (e.g. asbestos exposure is associated with pleural plaques, fibrosis and mesothelioma; isocyanite exposure with asthma). **Environmental** factors may be important (e.g. pet birds may cause psitticosis). **Travel** is associated with specific infections (e.g. Legionnaire's disease).

Examination (Fig. 19)

Detection of typical constellations of clinical signs helps establish a diagnosis, although poor inter-observer agreement questions their reliability and emphasizes the need for other investigations.

General examination

Determine if the patient is well or unwell and whether breathing, airway and circulation are adequate. Examine breathing rate and pattern. Assess the degree of breathlessness at rest or while undressing. Check observation charts (e.g. temperature, Sao_2) and bedside sputum pots. Note general features such as obesity, cachexia, jaundice, respiratory distress, anxiety and pain. Examine:

- *Hands:* for nicotine staining, finger clubbing (Fig 19; Table 1), peripheral cyanosis, the fine tremor of excessive B_2-agonist therapy and the coarse tremor of a CO_2 retention flap. A 'bounding' pulse also suggests CO_2 retention.
- *Face and neck:* for lymph nodes and features of systemic diseases. Examine the conjunctiva for anaemia and the tongue (lips) for central cyanosis (blue discoloration due to an increase in deoxygenated arterial haemoglobin). Measure the jugular venous pressure (JVP) and changes with respiration (i.e. fixed and raised in superior vena cava (SVC) obstruction). Check for tracheal deviation and stridor (inspiratory wheeze due to upper airway obstruction).

Chest examination

Includes anterior and posterior inspection, palpation, percussion and auscultation, with comparison of the left and right sides. The pattern of physical signs will indicate likely diagnoses (Table 2).

- *Inspection:* includes chest and spinal shape, scars of previous radiotherapy or surgery, subcutaneous nodules, engorged chest wall veins (SVC obstruction), hyperinflation, symmetry of chest wall movement and use of accessory muscles of respiration.
- *Palpation:* examine for tenderness, apex beat position and adequate chest wall expansion (>3 cm).
- *Percussion:* assess for dullness and hyper-resonance.
- *Auscultation:* assess breath sounds and their distribution including nature (i.e. vesicular, bronchial), intensity (i.e. absent, diminished) and added sounds (wheezes, crackles, rub). **'Vesicular' breath sounds** are normal inspiratory and expiratory sounds; there is no gap between inspiration and expiration. **Bronchial breath sounds** are high-pitched ('blowing') sounds with a gap between inspiration and expiration. They occur with consolidation, collapse and above pleural effusions. Reduced breath sounds occur with effusions, consolidation, pneumothorax and raised diaphragm. **Crepitations** may be fine, fixed and inspiratory due to pulmonary fibrosis or early consolidation; or coarse due to excessive bronchial secretions (e.g. bronchiectasis). **Vocal resonance** and **tactile vocal fremitus** increase over areas of consolidation and diminish over effusions and collapsed lung.

(a) Volume–time spirograms during forced expiration from total lung capacity

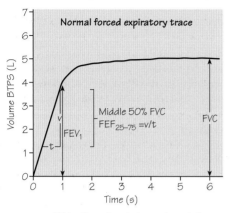

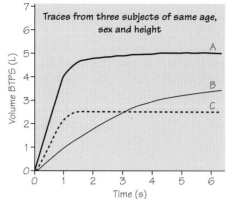

FEV$_1$ = Forced expiratory volume in 1s
FVC = Forced vital capacity
FEF$_{25-75}$ = Mean forced expiratory flow from 25–75% of FVC

A = Normal respiratory system
B = Obstructive airway disease
C = Restrictive lung disease

(b) Helium dilution for measuring functional residual capacity*

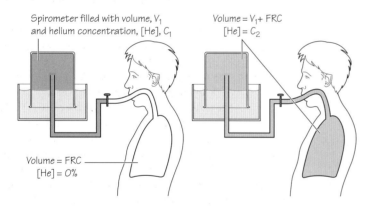

Spirometer filled with volume, V$_1$ and helium concentration, [He], C$_1$

Volume = V$_1$+ FRC
[He] = C$_2$

Volume = FRC
[He] = 0%

Starting at the end of a normal expiration (lung volume = FRC), the subject breathes in and out from the spirometer until equilibrium is reached. Since helium is poorly soluble in blood:

$$V_1 \times C_1 = (V_1 + FRC) \times C_2 \qquad \therefore FRC = V_1 \times \left(\frac{C_1 - C_2}{C_2} \right)$$

*Note: To measure TLC or RV the subject is asked to breathe in fully or breathe out fully before breathing the helium gas mixture.

(c) The body plethysmograph for measuring lung volumes

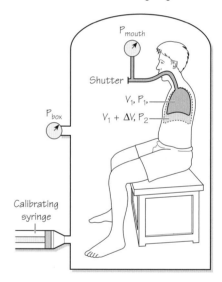

The subject inhales against a closed shutter

Lung volume expands from V$_1$ to V$_1$ + ΔV

ΔV can be deduced from the rise in box pressure, P$_{box}$ (calibrated with known volumes)

Mouth (= alveolar) pressure fall from P$_1$ to P$_2$

From Boyle's law: $V_1 \times P_1 = P_2(V_1 + \Delta V)$

Hence the original volume in the lungs, V$_1$ can be found

Accurate assessment of defects in airflow, lung volume or gas exchange is essential to the diagnosis and management of many respiratory disorders. It is important to note that these tests characterize 'defects'; the clinician has to diagnose 'diseases'. The normal range of many lung function tests is very wide and it is essential to compare measured values with those predicted for the subject's age, height and sex by standard **nomograms** derived from large cross-sectional studies.

Airway resistance can be measured using a **body plethysmograph** (Chapter 7; Fig. 20c) to measure alveolar pressure. **Lung compliance** can be measured using an **oesophageal balloon** to measure intrapleural pressure (for details see Chapter 6). More commonly, abnormalities of airway resistance (in obstructive airway disease) are assessed indirectly from forced expiratory manoeuvres and abnormalities of compliance (in restrictive lung disease) are assessed indirectly from lung volume measurements.

Forced expiratory tests

Peak expiratory flow rate (PEFR) is frequently measured, despite its inability to distinguish between different types of ventilatory defect and its dependence on patient effort (Fig. 7c). It is reduced in obstructive disease, respiratory muscle weakness and often in restrictive lung disease (secondary to reduced volume). Its main value lies in monitoring diseases, especially asthma, once the diagnosis has been made.

In contrast, plots of **volume against time (spirogram)** or **airflow against volume** during a forced expiration can help to distinguish between different types of defects. The patient is asked to inhale to total lung capacity (TLC) and breathe out as hard and fast as possible to residual volume (RV). A plot of volume against time (Fig. 20a) can be produced by continuously measuring volume, either with a spirometer or by integrating a flowmeter output. If a flowmeter is used, it is also possible to compute a flow–volume plot from the same forced expiration (Fig. 7c). Flow–volume plots show characteristic shapes with different defects (Fig. 7e), such as the 'scooped out' appearance seen in obstructive airway disease.

Forced vital capacity (FVC) and **forced expiratory volume in 't' seconds (FEV$_t$)** can be read off the volume–time plot (Fig. 20a). **FEV$_1$** is extremely reproducible and correlates well with function and prognosis. It is normal for FVC and FEV$_1$ to peak in adults in the third decade and then decline by approximately 30 mL/year (Chapter 38). Forced expiratory ratio (**FER = FEV$_1$/FVC**) is normally 0.75–0.90, but higher values may occur in normal children. FEV$_1$/FVC helps distinguish between obstructive and restrictive ventilatory defects. Typically, in obstructive lung diseases (e.g. COPD, acute asthma) the FEV$_1$/FVC is less than 0.70. If the airway obstruction is due to asthma, FEV$_1$, FVC and FEV$_1$/FVC may all increase after the inhalation of bronchodilators. In restrictive lung disease (e.g. lung fibrosis), absolute values of FEV$_1$ and FVC are reduced, but FEV$_1$/FVC is normal or high.

Forced mid-expiratory flow (FEF$_{25-75}$) is the average forced expiratory flow rate over the middle 50% of the FVC. It may be especially affected by small airway disease, but the normal range is wide.

Maximal voluntary ventilation (MVV) is measured by asking the subject to breathe as hard and fast as possible into a spirometer for 15 s, with the ventilation expressed in L/min. It is very dependent on effort and not very reproducible, but it may correlate well with subjective dyspnoea.

Lung volumes

Restrictive ventilatory defects (RVDs) are characterized by a reduction in TLC. Lung volumes such as TLC, RV and FRC can be measured by **helium dilution** (Fig. 20b) or by **body plethysmography** (Fig. 20c). The gas dilution method is simpler for patients, but it is sensitive to gas leaks and will underestimate TLC in the presence of extensive bullous or cystic lung disease. RVDs may be caused by parenchymal lung disease (pulmonary fibrosis, scleroderma, pulmonary oedema), chest wall disease (kyphoscoliosis, massive obesity) or weak respiratory muscles (myasthenia gravis, muscular dystrophy). RV and FRC can help distinguish between these conditions, as FRC and RV are usually reduced in lung disease; whereas FRC is usually normal and RV elevated in muscle weakness. FVC and TLC usually decline in parallel, therefore once an RVD has been established by measurement of TLC, the progress of the disease may be followed with FVC from spirometry.

Measurement of lung compliance (Chapter 6) and **transdiaphragmatic pressure** (P_{di}) may distinguish further between RVD due to parenchymal lung disease or muscle weakness. By using two small balloon-tipped catheters, one measuring oesophageal ($P_{pleural}$) pressure and the other gastric (P_{abd}) pressure, P_{di} ($= P_{abd} - P_{pleural}$) can be measured during a maximal inspiration or sniff from FRC. Typically, in parenchymal lung disease lung compliance is low, elastic recoil pressure high and P_{di} normal; whereas in respiratory muscle weakness lung compliance is relatively normal, elastic recoil pressure low, and P_{di} low.

Diffusing capacity, D_L (= transfer factor, T_L) is a measure of the ability of gas to diffuse from the alveolus into pulmonary capillary blood. As discussed in Chapter 5, D_LCO is used as a surrogate for D_LO_2, since it is simple to measure and carbon monoxide diffuses across the lung in a fashion similar to oxygen. It often helps interpretation to normalize D_LCO to the alveolar volume ($\dot{V}_A$) by calculating the coefficient, $Kco = D_LCO/\dot{V}_A$. D_LCO is reduced by reduced alveolar surface area, thickened alveolar–capillary membrane, reduced capillary blood volume or anaemia. Reductions in the D_LCO can be caused by a variety of parenchymal diseases (idiopathic pulmonary fibrosis, emphysema, pneumonia) or vascular diseases (pulmonary hypertension, pulmonary oedema), such that the test is sensitive but not specific. Reductions in the D_LCO below 50% predicted for age, sex and height are often associated with oxygen desaturation during exercise. Severe reductions in D_LCO (<20% predicted) may result in resting hypoxaemia.

Arterial blood gases (P_aO_2, P_aCO_2 and pHa) and **arterial oxygen saturation** are important tests of respiratory system function and are discussed in Chapters 22 and 42.

Evaluation of the CXR includes all the following:

(1) Date: (2) Name:

(3) AP/PA: Is it AP (anteroposterior)
    or PA (posteroanterior)?
    (Heart size cannot be measured if AP)

(4) Is it well positioned? The trachea should be
    midway between clavicles

(5) Penetration: The disc spaces should be just
    visible through the cardiac shadows
    (underpenetrated = plethoric lungs
      overpenetrated = dark lungs)

(6) Soft tissues and breast shadows
    (mastectomy in a female)

(7) Right diaphragm 2 cm higher than left
    (raised when paralysed, flat in asthma/COPD)

(8) Check ribs for fractures, metastases

(9) Right heart border = right atrium

(10) Hilium = bronchi, arteries and veins

(11) Superior vena cava

(12) Aortic arch

(13) Left heart border = left ventricle

(14) Pulmonary vessels

(15) Trachea and main bronchi

(16) Lung fields

---

(1) Thoracic vertebral bodies

(2) Scapula

(3) Pulmonary trunk and hilium

(4) Descending aorta

(5) Head of clavicle

(6) Trachea

(7) Arch of aorta

(8) Ascending aorta

(9) Anterior space (thymus)

(10) Heart

(11) Sternum

(12) Diaphragm

---

(1) Oesophagus

(2) Right lung

(3) Right main bronchus

(4) Right pulmonary artery and branches

(5) Superior vena cava

(6) Ascending aorta

(7) Pulmonary trunk

(8) Mediastinum and heart

(9) Left pulmonary artery and branches

(10) Left main bronchus

(11) Left lung

(12) Descending aorta

Chest radiograph interpretation

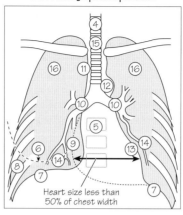

Heart size less than
50% of chest width

Chest radiograph interpretation

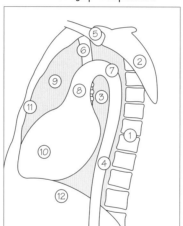

Normal chest X-ray

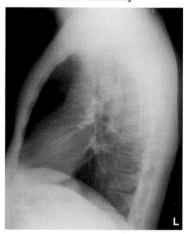

Normal lateral X-ray

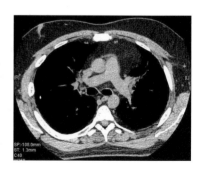

Standard (two-dimensional) chest X-rays: to detect, diagnose or follow morphological abnormalities in the chest are the mainstay of thoracic radiographical imaging and account for >50% of procedures. Recent innovations include digital, three-dimensional computed tomography (CT) scans and physiological (positron emission tomography, ventilation–perfusion scans) imaging. Specific radiographical abnormalities are discussed in individual chapters.

Posteroanterior (PA) and lateral chest radiographs (CXRs) allow two-dimensional visualization of the lungs, great vessels, heart, diaphragm and mediastinum. PA films should be performed upright in full inspiration. Routine lateral films are not required for screening purposes. Fig 19a illustrates CXR features and interpretation. Portable anterior–posterior films (AP) in patients unable to stand magnify the heart and mediastinum and do not allow detailed visualization of lung parenchyma.

A standard PA and lateral CXR should allow visualization of both lungs, including the diaphragmatic position, as well as the normal trachea, main carina, mainstem bronchi, major and minor fissures, aorta, main pulmonary arteries and heart. Understanding of the normal anatomy of a CXR is essential to allow recognition of abnormal lung parenchymal infiltrates, enlarged lymph nodes adjacent to the trachea or in the hila, enlarged pulmonary arteries, volume loss of a lobe or segment or cardiac enlargement. In the case of a suspected pleural effusion, lateral decubitus films allow visualization of as little as 50 mL of free-flowing fluid. Digital CXRs are being developed that allow more detailed views of the denser portions of the thorax and show finer detail of the lung parenchyma.

Computed tomography (CT): a limitation of standard CXR imaging is that the two-dimensional image obscures details and averages densities in the third dimension (anterior–posterior on the PA film). CT allows thin slice axial images and fine-detailed examination of intrathoracic structures. It is more sensitive at detecting small lesions and in determining their relationship to other intrathoracic structures. Gross features are shown in Fig. 19b. Indications for CT are:

- *Bronchial carcinoma:* to detect and assess operability and prognosis of tumours (Chapter 39) by determining location, size and the presence of abnormal lymph nodes (e.g. mediastinal, axillary)
- *Lung parenchymal disease:* to detect and localize interstitial lung infiltrates, bronchiectasis, cavities, bulla, fluid collections and airway abnormalities
- *Mediastinal masses:* to determine extent, relationship to other structures
- *Pleural disease:* to detect asbestos-related plaques, mesothelioma and to determine the cause of pleural effusions
- *Pulmonary emboli (PE):* administration of intravenous contrast allows imaging of the pulmonary blood vessels and detection of emboli

Examples of CT scans are shown in several chapters. Newer technology allows complete axial scanning of the thorax with a single breath-hold.

Ventilation–perfusion (V/Q) scans: are mostly performed in the evaluation of pulmonary embolism (Chapter 27). Gamma cameras can visualize radiopharmaceuticals either injected into the venous blood (perfusion) or inhaled (ventilation). Thromboembolism classically causes a V/Q mismatch, with absence of perfusion in the presence of ventilation. Unfortunately, the value of V/Q scans is limited by the observation that many PEs result in indeterminate V/Q scans that show small mismatches or matched V/Q deficits. In these cases, other studies must be utilized to demonstrate thromboemboli. Contrast CT scans are increasingly used to detect PE (see above) and are being investigated as possible replacements for V/Q scanning. Quantitative V/Q scans may be used in preparation for lung resection surgery, to assess regional lung function and estimate the amount of residual lung function.

Pulmonary angiography visualizes the vasculature following injection of contrast medium (Chapter 27). It may be required in patients with suspected pulmonary emboli but equivocal V/Q scans, pulmonary hypertension and pulmonary vascular disease, including vasculitis and arteriovenous malformations. These studies are often preceded by echocardiography to visualize right ventricular function and estimate pulmonary artery pressure using Doppler imaging.

Positron emission tomography (PET): utilizes a fluorinated analogue of glucose (FDG) to give images of the lung that highlight areas of increased glucose metabolism. Malignant cells have increased glucose uptake and appear as increased densities on PET images. Recent studies have demonstrated that PET is useful in distinguishing between benign and malignant solitary pulmonary nodules and in detecting small nodal metastases that are not detected on CT scanning. For these indications, PET has a sensitivity and specificity of 80–97% with false positive scans seen in cases of infection or granulomatous inflammation. Whole body PET was recently used to detect clinically inapparent distant metastases.

Bronchoscopy: enables direct visualization down to the 4th–5th division of the endobronchial tree. Chest physicians perform most bronchoscopies as day cases under local anaesthetic in the sedated but awake patient, using a flexible fibreoptic instrument. It has the advantages of visualization of the upper lobes and is a safe technique with a low complication rate. Saturation and heart rhythm should be monitored and supplemental oxygen administered during the procedure. Facilities for resuscitation should always be immediately available. Thoracic surgeons may use a rigid bronchoscope in the fully anaesthetized patient. This instrument allows larger biopsies and better suctioning, and is the method of choice when removing inhaled foreign bodies. Bronchoscopy is most frequently performed to investigate if a shadow on a chest radiograph is due to a lung cancer (Chapter 39). If an endobronchial tumour is seen, biopsies for histological analysis and washings and brush samples for cytological analysis can be taken. In addition, information regarding the operability of the tumour can be obtained. Bronchoscopy can also be used to diagnose parenchymal lung disease using the technique of transbronchial biopsy, which obtains parenchymal and bronchial tissue for histological examination. Collection of bronchoalveolar fluid (bronchoalveolar lavage, BAL) is useful in diagnosing alveolitis (raised lymphocyte count in sarcoidosis), infection in the immunocompromised patient (e.g. *Pneumocystis carinii* pneumonia) and tuberculosis. Bronchoscopy also aids investigation of collapsed segments or lobes. Therapeutically, bronchoscopy is used to remove inhaled foreign bodies, to aspirate sputum plugs and secretions, to relieve stenosis by placement of stents and during treatment of endobronchial tumours with laser or endobronchial radiotherapy. Haemorrhage, pneumothorax and cardiac arrhythmia, although uncommon, are the main complications of fibreoptic bronchoscopy.

22 Respiratory failure

(a) Causes of respiratory failure

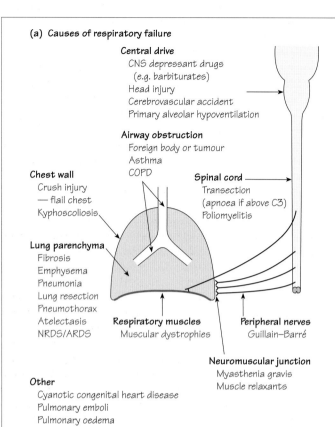

Central drive
CNS depressant drugs
  (e.g. barbiturates)
Head injury
Cerebrovascular accident
Primary alveolar hypoventilation

Airway obstruction
Foreign body or tumour
Asthma
COPD

Chest wall
Crush injury
  — flail chest
Kyphoscoliosis

Spinal cord
Transection
(apnoea if above C3)
Poliomyelitis

Lung parenchyma
Fibrosis
Emphysema
Pneumonia
Lung resection
Pneumothorax
Atelectasis
NRDS/ARDS

Respiratory muscles
Muscular dystrophies

Peripheral nerves
Guillain–Barré

Neuromuscular junction
Myasthenia gravis
Muscle relaxants

Other
Cyanotic congenital heart disease
Pulmonary emboli
Pulmonary oedema

(b) Mechanisms of arterial hypoxia (low P_aO_2)

Normal

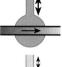

Normal alveolar-
capillary membrane

Normal P_IO_2

Normal alveolar ventilation

Normal P_aO_2

>98% cardiac
output passing
through gas-
exchanging alveoli

Matching of ventilation and perfusion
throughout the lungs

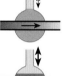

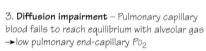

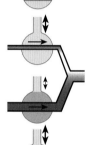

1. **Low inspired P_O_2** – e.g. altitude (low P_B) or low inspired O_2 concentration → low alveolar P_O_2

2. **Hypoventilation** – Inadequate alveolar ventilation → low alveolar P_O_2

3. **Diffusion impairment** – Pulmonary capillary blood fails to reach equilibrium with alveolar gas → low pulmonary end-capillary P_O_2

4. **Ventilation–perfusion mismatching** – Blood from areas with high $\dot{V}_A/\dot{Q}$ mixes with blood from low $\dot{V}_A/\dot{Q}$ areas → low pulmonary venous P_O_2

5. **Right-to-left shunt** – Shunted blood fails to undergo gas exchanges, mixes with pulmonary capillary blood → low pulmonary venous/left ventricular P_O_2

(c) Effects of hypoxia and hypercapnia

	Acute	Chronic—compensation and complications
Low P_aO_2 (hypoxaemia/ hypoxia)	**Impaired CNS function:** irritability, confusion, drowsiness, convulsions, coma, death **Central cyanosis** (not very sensitive; may be absent in anaemia) **Cardiac arrhythmias** **Hypoxic vasoconstriction*** of pulmonary vessels	**Erythropoietin** from hypoxic kidney → **polycythaemia** → ↑ oxygen carriage despite low P_aO_2 but if excessive (haematocrit >55%) the ↑viscosity impairs tissue blood flow **Polycythaemia** → florid complexion; increased cyanosis **Pulmonary hypertension*** → right ventricular hypertrophy **Fluid retention/right heart failure (cor pulmonale*)** → peripheral oedema/ascites/↑jugular venous pressure/enlarged liver
High P_aCO_2 (hypercapnia)	**Low arterial pH** (respiratory acidosis) **Peripheral vasodilatation** → warm flushed skin, bounding pulse **Cerebral vasodilatation** → ↑ intracranial pressure → headache, worse on waking if nocturnal ventilation↓ **Impaired CNS/muscle function:** irritability, confusion, somnolence, coma, tremor, myolonic jerks, hand flap **Cardiac arrhythmias**	**Renal compensation** (compensatory metabolic alkalosis) → ↑arterial $[HCO_3^-]$ → arterial pH returned to near normal **Cerebrospinal fluid (CSF) compensation** → ↑CSF $[HCO_3^-]$ → CSF pH returned to near normal → respiratory drive less at any given P_aCO_2 than in acute hypercapnia *Hypercapnia accentuates the effects of hypoxia on pulmonary blood vessels and therefore contributes to the development of cor pulmonale (see above)

Respiratory failure is usually said to exist when arterial P_{O_2} falls below 8 kPa (60 mmHg) when breathing air at sea level. In **type 1 respiratory failure**, the arterial hypoxia is accompanied by a normal or low arterial P_{CO_2}, whereas in **type 2 or ventilatory failure**, arterial P_{CO_2} is increased above 6.7 kPa (50 mmHg). Respiratory failure may be **acute** or **chronic**. In chronic respiratory failure, there are permanent abnormalities in blood gases, which typically worsen periodically (**acute on chronic**). This strict definition excludes some patients whose respiratory systems might otherwise be considered failing. Some patients have disabling **dyspnoea** (breathlessness) of respiratory origin but maintain $P_{O_2} > 8$ kPa.

Some of the many causes of respiratory failure are listed in Fig. 22a. Symptoms and signs clearly depend on the underlying cause. Dyspnoea and **tachypnoea** (increased respiratory rate) will be prominent in severe asthma but absent in conditions with reduced central drive.

Mechanisms leading to hypoxia and hypercapnia

Of the five causes of hypoxaemia (Fig. 22b), only **hypoventilation** inevitably causes increased $P_{a}CO_2$.

$$P_{a}CO_2 \propto \frac{\dot{V}CO_2}{\dot{V}_A} \text{ (Chapter 9)}$$

If hypoxia is out of proportion to the hypercapnia and the **A–a P_{O_2} gradient** (Chapter 14) is increased, one of the other mechanisms (3–5 in Fig. 20b) must also be present. The primary effect of **right-to-left shunts** and **ventilation–perfusion mismatching** is to raise arterial CO_2 content, but this is usually corrected or over-corrected by a reflex increase in ventilation (Chapters 13 & 14).

Thickening of the alveolar–capillary membrane in lung fibrosis may give rise to **diffusion impairment**, preventing equilibration of pulmonary capillary blood with alveolar gas, especially in exercise, when time in the capillary is reduced. However, in many conditions thought to cause diffusion impairment, there is also substantial V_A/Q mismatching, and this is probably the main cause of the hypoxia.

Effects of hypoxia and hypercapnia

The direct effects of hypoxia and hypercapnia, together with the compensations and complications that occur in chronic respiratory failure, are shown in Fig. 22c.

Although hypoxia usually offers the greatest threat to vital organs, hypercapnia and especially acidosis are also important and they often accentuate the adverse effects of each other. Hypoxia and hypercapnia are better tolerated when they develop slowly in chronic respiratory failure because of adaptations such as polycythaemia and compensatory metabolic alkalosis.

Cyanosis is a greyish-blue tinge seen when the microcirculation of a tissue contains a high concentration of deoxygenated haemoglobin. It may occur with impaired blood flow, for example in the hands and feet in circulatory shock, when it is known as **peripheral cyanosis**. When the arterial blood contains more than about 1.5–2 g/dL of deoxygenated haemoglobin, the concentration in the microcirculation reaches the critical level for cyanosis to be observable even in well-perfused tissues. This occurs with an arterial saturation of about 85% if haemo-globin concentration is normal (15 g/dL) and the resulting **central cyanosis** is visible in the tongue and mucus membranes of the mouth. It appears at higher oxygen saturations in polycythaemic patients, whereas in severe anaemia central cyanosis may be impossible, as it would require an O_2 saturation incompatible with life.

Respiratory failure in asthma

Hypoxia in a severe asthma attack is primarily due to V_A/Q mismatching. $P_{a}CO_2$ usually falls as the attack worsens, because peripheral chemoreceptor and pulmonary receptor stimulation produce a reflex increase in ventilation despite the increased work of breathing. A raised or even apparently normal $P_{a}CO_2$ (e.g. 5.3 kPa, 40 mmHg) in a severe hypoxic asthma attack is a cause for concern, as it may indicate the onset of exhaustion and potentially life-threatening asthma.

Respiratory failure in chronic obstructive pulmonary disease

The clinical picture of severe chronic obstructive pulmonary disease (COPD) is variable (Chapter 25), but two extreme patterns—the **pink puffer** (dyspnoea, no cyanosis at rest) and the **blue bloater** (cyanosis at rest, corpulmonale, oedema)—are recognized. The blue bloater is associated with type 2 respiratory failure. He or she has a chronically low $P_{a}O_2$ and high $P_{a}CO_2$ and these worsen with acute infections, which precipitate acute on chronic respiratory failure. Patients with chronic hypercapnia typically have a near-normal arterial pH owing to an efficient compensatory metabolic alkalosis via renal generation and retention of bicarbonate. During an acute exacerbation, $P_{a}CO_2$ may increase further and pH then falls significantly, as renal adjustments are slow. Arterial pH can therefore indicate the proportions of acute and chronic hypercapnia. Patients with chronic hypercapnia are at risk of respiratory depression and a further, potentially fatal, increase in $P_{a}CO_2$ if given high inspired oxygen (Chapter 42). This may be due to loss of hypoxic drive in the presence of reduced CO_2 sensitivity, but other mechanisms may contribute to the rise in $P_{a}CO_2$, including increased V_A/Q mismatching by the removal of hypoxic vasoconstriction. As these patients are on the steep part of the oxyhaemoglobin dissociation curve, significant improvements in arterial oxygen content can usually be achieved by small increases in $F_{I}O_2$ (to 24 or 28%). The resulting small improvement in $P_{a}O_2$ does not cause respiratory depression (Chapter 12).

Management

All patients suspected of having respiratory failure will need arterial blood gas measurement, as the severity is difficult to assess clinically. A chest X-ray helps detect possible causes and aggravating factors such as pneumonia or pneumothorax. Other investigations, including lung function tests, will depend on the clinical situation and likely underlying disease. Management will include airway maintenance, clearance of secretions, oxygen therapy (Chapter 42) and in some cases mechanical ventilation (Chapter 41). Specific therapies, such as bronchodilators and antibiotics, are directed at the underlying cause or aggravating factors. Abnormalities in haemoglobin concentration, fluid balance and cardiac output should be treated to improve tissue oxygen delivery and increase mixed venous oxygen content, which in turn will also reduce the effects of venous admixture on arterial oxygenation.

23 Asthma: pathophysiology

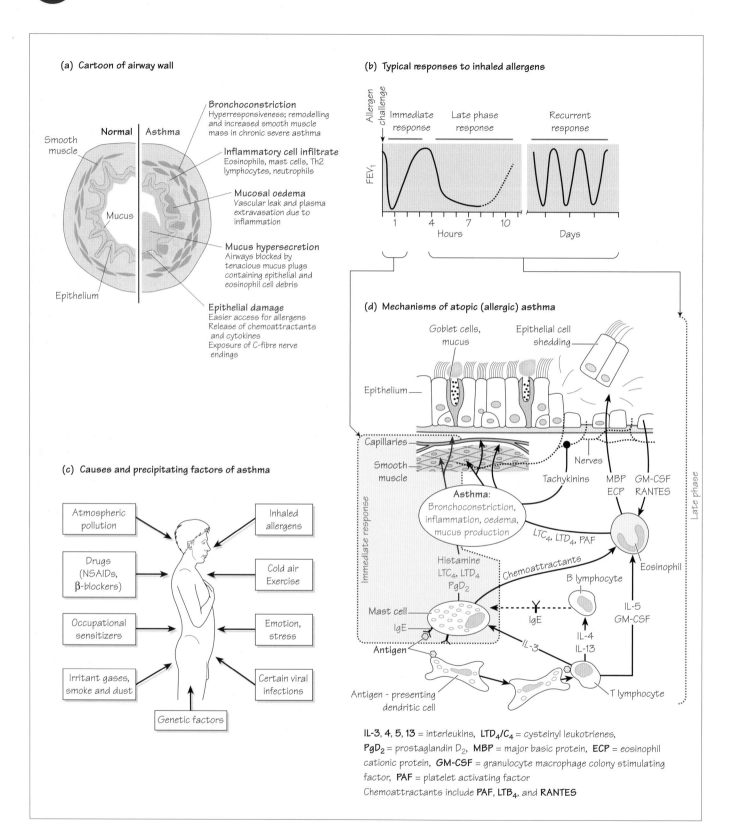

(a) Cartoon of airway wall

Bronchoconstriction
Hyperresponsiveness; remodelling and increased smooth muscle mass in chronic severe asthma

Inflammatory cell infiltrate
Eosinophils, mast cells, Th2 lymphocytes, neutrophils

Mucosal oedema
Vascular leak and plasma extravasation due to inflammation

Mucus hypersecretion
Airways blocked by tenacious mucus plugs containing epithelial and eosinophil cell debris

Epithelial damage
Easier access for allergens
Release of chemoattractants and cytokines
Exposure of C-fibre nerve endings

(b) Typical responses to inhaled allergens

(c) Causes and precipitating factors of asthma

Atmospheric pollution · Inhaled allergens · Drugs (NSAIDs, β-blockers) · Cold air Exercise · Occupational sensitizers · Emotion, stress · Irritant gases, smoke and dust · Certain viral infections · Genetic factors

(d) Mechanisms of atopic (allergic) asthma

IL-3, 4, 5, 13 = interleukins, LTD$_4$/C$_4$ = cysteinyl leukotrienes, PgD$_2$ = prostaglandin D$_2$, MBP = major basic protein, ECP = eosinophil cationic protein, GM-CSF = granulocyte macrophage colony stimulating factor, PAF = platelet activating factor
Chemoattractants include PAF, LTB$_4$, and RANTES

Asthma is an inflammatory disorder of the airways. Patients suffer from episodes of cough, wheezing, chest tightness and/or dyspnoea (breathlessness), which are often worse at night or early in the morning. There is considerable variation in the severity and frequency of attacks. Asthma can be usefully defined as '*increased responsiveness of the bronchi to various stimuli, manifested by widespread narrowing of the airways that changes in severity either spontaneously or as a result of treatment*'. The major characteristics of asthma are as follow (Fig. 23a):

1 **Narrowing of the airways** and impeded air flow, commonly reversible spontaneously or following treatment.

2 Increased sensitivity to bronchoconstricting stimuli (**hyperresponsiveness**).

3 Increased numbers of **inflammatory cells** (eosinophils, mast cells, neutrophils, T lymphocytes) in the bronchi.

There is also **hypersecretion of mucus**, blockage of airways with **mucus plugs** and swelling of mucosa due to inflammation-associated vascular leak and **oedema**, all of which further limit air flow. Damage to the epithelium (**epithelial shedding**) is reflected by whorls of epithelial cells (Curschmann's spirals) in the mucus, which also contains eosinophil cell membranes (Charcot–Leyden crystals). In chronic severe asthma, **remodelling of the airway wall** tissue structure occurs, including increased bronchial smooth muscle content. This causes irreversible narrowing of the airways and limits the effectiveness of bronchodilators.

Prevalence

Asthma is increasing in prevalence, particularly in the Western world, where >5% of the population may be symptomatic and receiving treatment. There has been a concomitant increase in mortality, despite improved treatment. In the UK, one in seven of the population has allergic disease and over 9 million people will have wheezed in the last year. The number of teenagers with asthma has nearly doubled over the last 12 years. Asthma is least common in the Far East and most common in the UK, Australia and New Zealand. There is some correlation with Westernized life-styles, including living conditions that favour house-dust mites and atmospheric pollution. Many factors can cause or precipitate asthma (Fig. 23c); 20% of the working population may be susceptible to occupational asthma (Chapter 31).

Classification

Asthma can be classified as **extrinsic**, having a definite external cause, and **intrinsic**, where no external cause can be identified. Extrinsic asthma commonly occurs as a result of an allergic response, with development of **IgE antibodies** to specific antigens (**allergic or atopic asthma**) and tends to start in childhood with symptoms becoming less severe with age; ~80% of asthmatics are atopic. Intrinsic asthma generally appears in adults and does not improve.

Atopic asthma

Individuals who readily produce IgE to common antigens are prone to allergic asthma. Major antigens include proteins in fecal pellets from **house-dust mite**—the most common cause of asthma worldwide—grass pollen and dander from **domestic pets**. Genetic factors, atmospheric pollution and maternal smoking in pregnancy all predispose to raised IgE levels and later development of asthma and airway hyperresponsiveness (Fig. 23a).

Inhalation of allergens by atopic individuals initiates an **immediate response** (bronchoconstriction) that usually subsides within 2 h (Fig. 23b); this is reversible with bronchodilators such as the β_2-adrenoceptor agonist salbutamol (Chapter 24). This is often followed 3–12 h later by a **late-phase response** with bronchoconstriction, airway inflammation and oedema, and hyperresponsiveness, which is less susceptible to bronchodilators. Some materials such as **isocyanates** cause only an **isolated late phase**. The increased hyperresponsiveness may promote **recurrent asthma attacks** over several days.

The immediate response is caused by antigen/IgE-induced **mast cell degranulation** and release of **histamine, prostaglandin D_2** (PgD_2) and **leukotriene C_4 and D_4** (LTC_4, LTD_4); these cause bronchoconstriction, increased mucus production and vascular leak (Fig. 23d). In the late phase, mediators from mast cells and activated **T lymphocytes** cause infiltration of **neutrophils** and **eosinophils**. Eosinophils are present in large numbers in asthmatic bronchi and release **leukotrienes**, platelet-activating factor (**PAF**), **major basic protein** (MBP) and **eosinophil cationic protein** (ECP). MBP and ECP contribute to epithelial cell damage, causing increased permeability to allergens, release of eosinophil chemoattractants (e.g. eotaxin, RANTES) and cytokines such as granulocyte macrophage colony-stimulating factor (GM-CSF), and exposure of C-fibre afferent nerve endings which release proinflammatory tachykinins.

Drug-associated asthma

Aspirin and other non-steroidal anti-inflammatory drugs (NSAIDs) promote asthmatic attacks in 5% of asthmatics. They inhibit the cyclo-oxygenase (COX) pathway that synthesizes prostaglandins and shift arachidonic acid metabolism from COX towards the lipoxygenase pathway and production of LTC_4 and LTD_4. Aspirin-induced asthma is partially reversed by antileukotriene therapy (Chapter 24).

The bronchi have little sympathetic innervation, but circulating epinephrine (adrenaline) acting via β_2-adrenoceptors on smooth muscle causes bronchodilatation. Consequently β-adrenoceptor antagonists such as propranolol can cause bronchoconstriction in asthmatics. This may even occur with nominally β_1-selective drugs and their use for cardiovascular disease should be avoided in asthmatics.

Other factors (Fig. 23b)

Asthmatics have hyperresponsive airways and irritants that do not affect healthy individuals can precipitate asthmatic attacks or worsen symptoms, for example **tobacco smoke** and **exhaust fumes** (Chapter 31). Exercise and inhalation of cold air often precipitate wheezing in asthmatics, probably via drying and cooling of the bronchial epithelium. This is common in children. Emotional stress can also induce an asthmatic attack. Certain **viral infections** (rhinovirus, parainfluenza, respiratory syncytial virus) are also associated with asthma attacks. It is also now believed that there is a genetic component to asthma.

24 **Asthma: treatment**

(a) Step-wise approach to asthma therapy

Step up: If control is not maintained, consider stepping up therapy,
but review avoidance of allergens and patient compliance

Step	Symptoms	Typical PEFR (% predicted)	Long-term control	Quick relief
1	Less frequent than daily	100%	None required	*For all stages:*
2	Daily	≤80%	Anti-inflammatory drugs: Low-dose inhaled steroids (<800 µg daily) Other controller drugs if steroids cannot be used	*Short-acting broncho-dilator as required (inhaled β_2-agonist)*
3	Moderate to severe	50–80%	Add long-acting β_2-agonists (salmeterol)	
4	Severe	50–80%	Add any or all of: (empirical trial) increased inhaled steroids to <2000 µg daily, oral β_2-agonists, theophylline, leukotriene receptor antagonists	*Used more than once daily or increasing use indicates need for additional long-term therapy*
5	Severe deteriorating	≤50%	Add oral prednisolone (40 mg daily)	
6	Further deterioration	≤30%	Hospitalization	

Based on British Thoracic Society Guidelines, Thorax 2002

Step down: Review treatment regime every 1–6 months; a gradual step-wise reduction in therapy may be possible

(b) Drugs used in asthma therapy

Type	β_2-adrenoreceptor agonists	Muscarinic receptor antagonists	Xanthines	Corticosteroids	Cromones	Anti-leukotrienes
	Inhaled, oral and IV: **Short acting:** Salbutamol (albuterol) Terbutaline, Rimeterol, Fenoterol, Pirbuterol **Long acting:** Salmeterol, Formoterol	*Inhaled:* Ipratropium bromide Oxitropium bromide	*Oral and IV:* Theophylline Aminophylline Enprofylline *Slow release preparations*	*Inhaled:* Beclometasone proprionate, Fluticasone proprionate, Budesonide *Oral:* Prednisone, Prednisolone *Intravenous:* Hydrocortisone Methylprednisolone	*Inhaled:* Sodium cromoglycate (cromolyn) Nedocromil sodium	*Oral:* **Receptor antagonists:** Montelukast, Pranlukast, Zafirlukast **Lipoxygenase inhibitors:** Zileuton
Adverse affects (dose related)	Muscle tremor (most common) Tachycardia, palpitations (less common) Hypokalaemia (?, high infused dose)	Rare Ipratropium – bitter taste	Headaches, nausea, vomiting, abdominal discomfort, diuresis, cardiac arrhythmias, epilepsy, behavioural disturbance (?) Interactions with many drugs affect plasma levels; important due to narrow therapeutic range	*Inhaled:* Oral candidiasis, hoarseness, cough *Oral and high dose:* Growth retardation, bruising, suppression of hypothalamic-pituitary axis, osteoporosis, water retention, hypertension, weight gain, eye problems, diabetes, psychosis	Rare Throat irritation with inhaled powder	None significant described so far, though zafirlukast has been associated with some cases of Churg–Strauss syndrome, a very rare vasculitis. These cases may however be related to a reduced steroid dose rather than the drug dose itself

(c) Pressurized metered dose inhaler

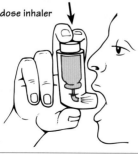

- Remove the cap and shake the inhaler
- Tilt the head back slightly and exhale
- Position the inhaler in the mouth (or preferably just in front of the open mouth)
- During a slow inspiration, press down the inhaler to release the medication
- Continue inhalation to full inspiration
- Hold breath for 10 seconds
- Actuate only one puff per inhalation

56 **Diseases and treatment** Asthma: treatment

Management of asthma should encompass: assessment of severity and efficacy of therapy; identification and removal of precipitating factors; therapy to reverse bronchoconstriction and inflammation; patient and family participation and education.

Assessment

Lung function: Asthma is diagnosed when inhaled bronchodilators cause >15% improvement in forced expiratory volume in 1 second (FEV_1) or peak expiratory flow rate (PEFR) (Chapter 20). The absence of improvement does not rule out asthma—the patient could be in remission and chronic severe asthma is poorly reversible. Airway resistance is least at midday and greatest at 3–4 a.m. Serial measurements of PEFR in the morning, midday and on retiring are useful for identifying the enhanced variation in airflow limitation characteristic of asthma and for assessing response to therapy over time. Poorly controlled asthma shows a characteristic morning fall in PEFR ('**morning dipping**'). Occupational asthma is suggested when PEFR improves after a break from work. Lung function tests are often coupled with exercise tests in children, who often exhibit exercise-induced asthma.

Bronchial provocation tests are used to determine hyperresponsiveness when asthma is suspected but PEFR measurements are not diagnostic. Patients inhale increasing doses of histamine or methacholine (acetylcholine analogue) until FEV_1 declines by 20%. The dose at which this occurs ($PD_{20}FEV_1$) is greatly reduced in asthmatics, who are always hyperresponsive.

Skin prick tests identify extrinsic factors. Development of a wheal around the prick site indicates allergen sensitivity. Exposure to identified allergens should be immediately minimized (e.g. replacement of furnishings to reduce house-dust mite; removal of pets), as once extrinsic asthma is established it may not be reversible. Only 50% of patients with occupational asthma are cured by avoidance of the precipitating factor.

Therapy

The goal is long-term control and all patients except those with the mildest symptoms should receive anti-inflammatory drugs as well as bronchodilators. International guidelines favour **step-wise treatment regimens** (Fig. 24a). Asthma therapy is centred on **inhaled** compounds (Fig. 24b). Inhalation maximizes bronchial delivery while minimizing systemic side-effects. Metered dose inhalers are the most commonly used delivery systems, although only ~15% of the dose may reach the lungs (Fig. 24c).

β_2-Adrenoceptor agonists such as salbutamol are rapid and powerful bronchodilators and are of first choice for alleviating acute symptoms. They activate adenylate cyclase to increase cyclic adenosine monophosphate (cAMP) and may also reduce mediator release from inflammatory cells and airway nerves. Long-acting β_2-agonists such as salmeterol allow twice-daily dosage regimens. Long-term use of β_2-agonists is associated with reduced effectiveness (**tolerance**).

Muscarinic receptor antagonists (ipratropium) block the effects of acetylcholine from parasympathetic nerves, and are moderately effective bronchodilators and reduce mucus secretion. They are more effective against irritants than allergens. May be additive to β_2-agonists.

Corticosteroids such as beclometasone are the most important anti-inflammatory drugs. They reduce eosinophil numbers and activation and activity of macrophages and lymphocytes. **Inhaled corticosteroids** are the mainstay of long-term asthma therapy. However, they can have significant side-effects, including oral candidiasis (5%) and

hoarseness. Growth may be retarded in children receiving high-dose inhaled corticosteroids. **Oral corticosteroids** such as prednisolone may be required in patients whose asthma cannot be controlled by inhaled steroids, but the danger of adverse effects is much greater. **Combination therapies** containing both steroid plus long-acting β_2-agonists are useful for moderate/severe asthmatics.

Cromoglycate and **nedocromil** inhibit release of inflammatory mediators and prevent activation of mast cells and eosinophils. They may also suppress sensory nerve activity and release of neuropeptides (Chapter 23). Although of no value in acute attacks, prophylactic use reduces both immediate and late phases of the asthmatic response and hyperresponsiveness. Less powerful than steroids, they are only effective in mild and exercise-induced asthma. However, they have few side-effects and are often the drug of choice for children. Use has declined since the introduction of safer, low-dose steroids, which are cheaper, more effective and do not need to be taken so often.

Xanthines such as theophylline have bronchodilatory and some anti-inflammatory actions and are taken orally. They inhibit phosphodiesterases that break down cAMP. Limitations include numerous side-effects and a narrow therapeutic range; these are partially overcome by slow-release preparations. Xanthines are used as second-line drugs in asthma, particularly where β_2-agonists are ineffective at controlling symptoms and in steroid-resistant asthma.

Anti-leukotriene therapy comes in two forms: cysLT receptor (LTC_4/D_4) antagonists such as montelukast, and 5-lipoxygenase inhibitors such as zileuton. Both have equal efficacy for bronchoconstriction caused by allergens, exercise and cold air, with ~50% reversal. They are effective in aspirin-sensitive asthma, indicating the key role leukotrienes have in this condition (Chapter 23). Anti-leukotrienes improve lung function in mild and moderate asthmatics, but the greatest benefit may be for very severe asthmatics taking steroids. Both drug types are taken orally and are relatively long-lasting, with few adverse effects.

Histamine antagonists have not proved useful in asthma, although newer, non-sedating antihistamines such as terfenadine may alleviate mild allergic asthma.

Novel therapies: recombinant anti-IgE antibody (omalizumab) has been shown to be effective in moderate to severe allergic asthma, by reducing levels of antigen-specific IgE. Anti-cytokine antibodies (e.g. anti-IL-13) are in development, but not proven.

Problems with treatment

Failure to control asthma is often related to poor compliance with treatment regimens—for example, due to peer pressure in children. Compliance may also be poor when asthma is apparently controlled, so patients stop therapy (e.g. steroids, cromoglycate) because they are 'cured'. Poor inhaler techniques are common. Patient education and training is key to asthma therapy.

Severe uncontrolled asthma—'status asthmaticus'

This requires immediate treatment and hospitalization. **Indications:** inability to complete sentences ('telegraph speaking'), high respiratory rate, tachycardia, PEFR <50% predicted.

Dangerously life-threatening when bradycardia/hypotension, cyanosis or coma/exhaustion are present and/or PEFR <30% predicted. **Treatment:** immediate nebulized β_2-agonists delivered in oxygen and intravenous steroids, with subsequent oral prednisolone. In unresolving cases, intravenous β_2-agonists or xanthines and ventilation may be required.

25 Chronic obstructive pulmonary disease

(a) Risk factors for COPD

Smoking
Age >50 years
Male
Childhood chest infections
Airway hyperreactivity (asthma)
Low socioeconomic status
α_1-antitrypsin deficiency
Atmospheric pollution

(b) Spirometry in COPD

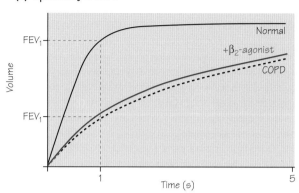

Normal: $FEV_1/FVC > 0.8$; **COPD**: $FEV_1/FVC < 0.7$;
Bronchodilator has <15% improvement (i.e. irreversible)

(c) Pathophysiology of COPD

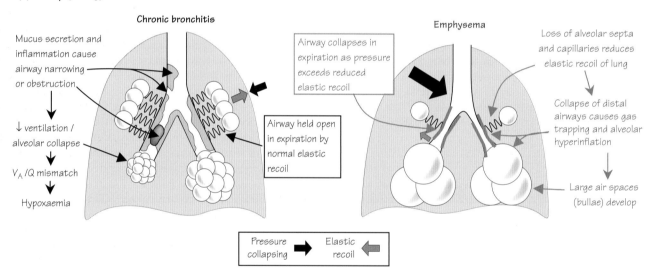

Chronic bronchitis

Mucus secretion and inflammation cause airway narrowing or obstruction

$\downarrow$ ventilation / alveolar collapse

V_A/Q mismatch

Hypoxaemia

Airway collapses in expiration as pressure exceeds reduced elastic recoil

Airway held open in expiration by normal elastic recoil

Emphysema

Loss of alveolar septa and capillaries reduces elastic recoil of lung

Collapse of distal airways causes gas trapping and alveolar hyperinflation

Large air spaces (bullae) develop

Pressure collapsing ➡ Elastic recoil ⬅

(d) Typical signs and symptoms of COPD

Chronic bronchitis	Emphysema
Chronic cough, producing sputum Hypoventilation, little respiratory effort Cyanosis, hypoxaemia with secondary polycythaemia CO_2 retention/chronic hypercapnia 　– leading to peripheral vasodilatation and bounding pulse Oedema Cor pulmonale **Normal** lung volumes, D_LCO, lung compliance	Chronic breathlessness (dyspnoea) Cyanosis unusual; normoxic at rest, hypoxic on exercise Barrel chest (hyperinflation), underweight Rarely exhibit oedema or cor pulmonale **Increased** TLC, RV, lung compliance **Reduced** D_LCO
Note: Most patients may present with both chronic bronchitis and emphysema	

Chronic obstructive pulmonary disease (COPD) is characterized by irreversible expiratory airflow obstruction and increased work of breathing. Other terms are COLD and COAD (chronic obstructive lung/airway disease). COPD encompasses **chronic bronchitis** and **emphysema**, which often present together. Typically, smoking and other risk factors (Fig. 25a) accelerate the normal age-related decline in lung function (Chapter 38), and cause chronic respiratory symptoms interposed with intermittent **acute exacerbations**, eventually leading to disability and **respiratory failure** (Chapter 22). Chronic hypoxaemia in COPD can lead to **pulmonary hypertension** (Chapter 26). Asthma is not classified as COPD as it is reversible (Chapters 23 & 24).

Diagnosis and pathophysiology

COPD is diagnosed by airflow obstruction indicated by a **reduced FEV_1/FVC ratio** of <0.7 which is irreversible (<15% increase in FEV_1) with bronchodilator or steroid therapy (Fig. 25b; Chapter 20). Restrictive lung disease (e.g. fibrosis) should be excluded. Patients with COPD have symptoms of **dyspnoea** (breathlessness) at rest or on exertion. Many asymptomatic smokers have lung function abnormalities that predate symptoms, which may be prevented by early smoking cessation. Although chronic bronchitis and emphysema most often coexist, they reflect different underlying processes (Fig. 25c) with differing signs and symptoms (Fig. 25d).

Chronic bronchitis is associated with airways obstruction caused by **chronic mucosal inflammation**, **mucous gland hypertrophy** and mucus **hypersecretion**, coupled with **bronchospasm** (Fig. 25c). It is defined by daily morning cough and excessive mucus production for 3 months in 2 successive years, in the absence of airway tumour, acute/chronic infection or uncontrolled cardiac disease. Most patients have normal total lung capacity (TLC), functional residual capacity (FRC), residual volume (RV), $D_L CO$ (diffusing capacity) and static lung compliance (Chapter 20). Patients with advanced chronic bronchitis have reduced respiratory drive and CO_2 **retention**, which is associated with bounding pulse, vasodilatation, confusion, headache, flapping tremor and papilloedema. **Hypoxaemia** is mostly due to V_A/Q mismatch (Fig. 25c; Chapter 14), and leads to **polycythaemia** (increased red cells) and **increased pulmonary artery pressure** (pulmonary hypertension) due to **hypoxic pulmonary vasoconstriction**. The resulting impairment of right heart function leads to renal fluid retention, raised central venous pressure and **peripheral oedema**, subsequently leading to **cor pulmonale** (fluid retention/heart failure secondary to lung disease). Pulmonary hypertension is potentiated by extensive capillary loss in late disease. There are no radiographical signs diagnostic of chronic bronchitis.

Emphysema is caused by **progressive destruction of alveolar septa** and capillaries, leading to development of **enlarged airways and airspaces** (bullae), **decreased lung elastic recoil** and **increased airway collapsibility**. Airways obstruction is caused by collapse of distal airways during expiration due to loss of elastic radial traction present in the normal lung (Fig. 25c). The resulting **hyperinflation** enhances expiratory airflow but inspiratory muscles work at a mechanical disadvantage. The pathophysiology of emphysema may involve an imbalance between inflammatory cell proteases and anti-protease defences (Chapter 18). Centrilobular emphysema is associated with cigarette smoking and predominantly involves the upper lung zones. Panacinar emphysema is associated with α_1-**antitrypsin deficiency** (Chapter 18) and predominantly involves the lower lung zones. Patients with emphysema typically have airflow obstruction with **elevated TLC, FRC** and **RV, reduced $D_L CO$** and **increased static lung compliance**. Such patients tend to be breathless and **tachypnoeic** (fast respiratory rate) at rest, with signs of hyperinflation and malnutrition including barrel chest and thin body, use of accessory respiratory muscles and **purse-lipped breathing**. The latter increases pressure in the upper airways and thus limits distal airway collapse. Auscultation reveals distant breath sounds with a prolonged expiratory wheeze. Blood gases are normal at rest, with marked O_2 desaturation during exertion. Radiographically, emphysema may appear as hyperinflated lungs with a large retrosternal airspace and flat diaphragms. When the condition is advanced, there may be areas with a lack of vascularity or visualization of bullae. High-resolution computed tomography (CT) is useful to demonstrate enlarged airspaces and air trapping.

Management

No specific therapy reverses COPD but treatment can slow disease progression, ease chronic symptoms and prevent acute exacerbations. Smoking cessation is critical.

β-Agonists (salbutamol) and **anticholinergics** may improve symptoms and lung function, possibly having additive effects when combined. **Theophylline** has negligible effects on spirometry, yet may improve exercise performance and blood gases. Patients producing large amounts of sputum may benefit from **mucolytics**. Oral **corticosteroids** (to reduce inflammation) improve function in less than 25% of COPD patients, but side-effects limit use. Inhaled corticosteroids may be considered in severe disease ($FEV_1 < 1$ L). **Pulmonary rehabilitation** strengthens respiratory muscles and improves quality of life and exercise tolerance while reducing hospitalizations; it has no effect on lung function. O_2 **therapy** prolongs life in patients with resting daytime hypoxaemia by slowing progression of cor pulmonale. O_2 should be utilized as much as possible, as benefit increases with use. Patients with nocturnal or exercise desaturation benefit from supplemental O_2 at night or during exercise. In α_1-**antitrypsin deficiency**, replacement therapy can increase plasma and lung antiprotease levels; however, the benefits on lung function and survival are controversial. Surgical **lung volume reduction** or **transplantation** may be indicated in advanced COPD, but long-term efficacy has not been established.

Prevention of acute COPD exacerbations include pneumococcal and influenza vaccination. Patients with any combination of increased dyspnoea, increased sputum or purulent sputum benefit from antibiotics targeted against common respiratory pathogens (*Haemophilus influenzae, Moraxella catarrhalis, Streptococcus pneumoniae*). Short courses of oral corticosteroids improve lung function and hasten recovery in patients with acute exacerbations.

Overall prognosis for COPD patients is dependent on the severity of airflow obstruction. Patients with a $FEV_1 < 0.8$ L have a yearly mortality of ~25%. Patients with cor pulmonale, hypercapnia, ongoing cigarette smoking and weight loss have a worse prognosis. Death usually occurs from infection, acute respiratory failure, pulmonary embolus or cardiac arrhythmia.

(a) Causes of pulmonary hypertension (World Health Organisation classification)

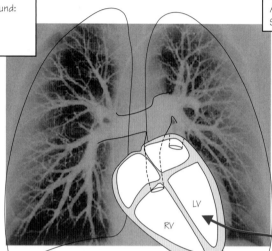

Pulmonary arterial hypertension:
Idiopathic pulmonary arterial vasculopathy (PAV)
Persistent PH of the newborn
Familial PH
Associated with PH, but no causal link found:
- Collagen vascular disease
- HIV
- Portal hypertension

Secondary to respiratory disease:
Alveolar hypoxia -
COPD (Chapter 25)
Interstitial lung disease (Chapter 29)
ARDS (Chapter 40)
Sleep-disordered breathing (Chapter 43)

Secondary to thrombotic disease:
Chronic thromboembolic disease
Embolic obliterative disease

**Disorders directly affecting
the vasculature:**
Interstitial lung disease (Chapter 29)
Vasculitis (Chapter 28)
Emphysema (Chapter 25)
Schistosomiasis

Pulmonary venous hypertension:
Left ventricular heart failure
Mitral stenosis/insufficiency
Fibrosing mediastinitis
Left atrial myxoma
Veno-occlusive disease

(b) Evaluation of suspected pulmonary hypertension

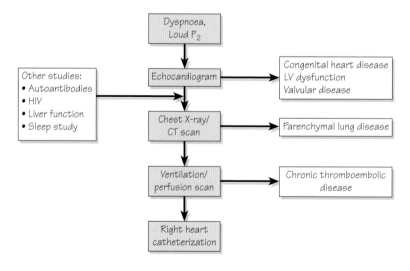

Dyspnoea,
Loud P_2

Other studies:
• Autoantibodies
• HIV
• Liver function
• Sleep study

Echocardiogram → Congenital heart disease / LV dysfunction / Valvular disease

Chest X-ray/ CT scan → Parenchymal lung disease

Ventilation/ perfusion scan → Chronic thromboembolic disease

Right heart catheterization

Pulmonary hypertension (PH) is defined as a systolic pulmonary arterial (PA) pressure >**30 mmHg** or mean PA pressure >**25 mmHg** (normal values: ~20 mmHg systolic, ~14 mmHg mean). Although common, its aetiology may be complex because it can be caused by many kinds of abnormality. This is because PA pressure is a function of **pulmonary vascular resistance**, **cardiac output** and **back-pressure** (left atrial pressure), all of which may be altered by multifarious factors. Most commonly PH is caused by another disorder (**secondary PH**). Much more rarely there is no apparent cause (**idiopathic pulmonary arterial vasculopathy** (PAV) or **primary PH**). Development of PH can substantially increase morbidity and mortality, and patients usually die from **progressive right heart failure**. Chronic PH can lead to **remodelling** and thickening of the pulmonary vasculature, reducing the efficacy of vasodilators.

PH is generally slow to develop and presents with non-specific symptoms, including dyspnoea on exertion, shortness of breath, palpitations, chest pain, light-headedness and syncope. Signs are difficult to elicit early and may only include an increased pulmonic component of the second heart sound. With more severe hypertension, **right ventricular dysfunction** will be apparent, including jugular venous distension, right ventricular heave, pedal oedema and hepatic enlargement. Detection of PH requires a high index of suspicion, because signs and symptoms are non-specific and the diagnosis requires further testing; there is significant under-diagnosis.

Types of pulmonary hypertension

Secondary to respiratory disease: most common, due to hypoxaemia which causes small pulmonary arteries to constrict (**hypoxic pulmonary vasoconstriction**). PH is often associated with COPD (Chapter 25). Any condition leading to hypoxia can cause PH, including sleep-disordered breathing (Chapter 43) and exposure to altitude.

Pulmonary venous hypertension: increased left atrial (LA) pressure, most commonly due to left ventricular dysfunction as in **congestive heart failure**, leads to elevation of PA pressure by increasing back-pressure through the lungs. **Mitral insufficiency** or **stenosis** may also increase PA pressure enough to cause hypertension. In these cases, patients will often have signs of pulmonary capillary hypertension such as crackles. Echocardiography should demonstrate LA enlargement.

Secondary to thrombotic disease: acute and chronic venous **thromboembolism** causes PH by mechanical obstruction of the proximal or distal pulmonary arteries. In acute thromboembolism, a component of vasospasm is also present, as the platelet-rich thromboembolus releases vasoactive mediators such as thromboxane, serotonin or platelet-activating factor. This form is also associated with sickle cell disease.

Disorders directly affecting the vasculature: increases in pulmonary vascular resistance may occur in the veins, capillaries or arteries. Increases in **capillary resistance** are common and may occur in any lung disease that causes capillary distortion or reduction in surface area. **Interstitial lung diseases** (Chapter 29) such as pulmonary **fibrosis**, **scleroderma** or **sarcoidosis** cause capillary distortion, as lung parenchyma is affected. Destruction of capillaries occurs in **emphysema** (Chapter 25) or pneumonectomy. In schistosomiasis (bilharzia) the parasitic worms can block pulmonary capillaries.

Pulmonary arterial hypertension includes PAV, PH associated with conditions such as collagen vascular disease, HIV and portal hypertension but where no causal relationship can be determined, and persistent pulmonary hypertension of the newborn (PPHN). PAV is rare (1–2 per million population) and its pathogenesis unclear. Genetic abnormalities, in particular related to bone morphogenic protein and serotonin transporters, may predispose patients to PAV, but although some cases are clearly **familial** with autosomal dominant inheritance, other are **sporadic** with no family history. PAV is more common in women than men (ratio 1.7 : 1) and most prevalent between 20–40 years of age. Certain appetite-suppressant drugs affecting serotonin (e.g. flenfluramine) are associated with a 30-fold increase in risk after 3 months. Remodelling of pulmonary arterioles is characteristic of PAV, although in some patients a component of arterial vasospasm is suggested by the effect of vasodilators. PAV may be associated with autoimmune diseases such as scleroderma.

Evaluation

Evaluation of patients with suspected PH (Fig. 26b) begins with **echocardiography**, allowing calculation of right ventricular systolic pressure and visualization of left atrium (LA), mitral valve, right ventricle and congenital abnormalities. If PH is found in conjunction with an enlarged LA, it is most likely due to either left ventricular or mitral disease. Chest radiology, pulmonary function testing and measurement of arterial oxygen allow detection of parenchymal disease or hypoxia. In the absence of LA enlargement or pulmonary parenchymal disease, further evaluation of pulmonary arteries is necessary. Ventilation/perfusion scanning is most useful to demonstrate chronic thromboemboli (Chapter 27). **Right heart catheterization** is the definitive test for the assessment of PH, as PA pressure can be measured directly and LA pressure estimated from the pulmonary capillary wedge pressure. Patients with PH without an elevated LA pressure and no apparent pulmonary venous, lung parenchymal, chronic thromboemboli or congenital heart disease are assumed to have PAV.

Management

Therapy in most patients is directed at the underlying abnormality, to relieve right ventricular strain and prevent right heart failure. There is generally no specific therapy for PH in cases of left ventricular dysfunction, pulmonary venous disease or pulmonary parenchymal diseases. Hypoxaemic patients with COPD benefit from O_2 therapy to diminish hypoxic vasoconstriction. Patients with **thromboembolic disease** (Chapter 27) should receive anticoagulation and evaluation for surgical thromboembolectomy. Patients with PAV should also receive **anticoagulation** to prevent microthrombi or the devastating effect of an acute thromboembolus (Chapter 27). Most patients with PAV require chronic infusions or nebulization of **prostacyclin** analogues to improve survival. Prostacyclin has acute vasodilator properties, but an effect on pulmonary vascular remodelling or endothelial function may explain its positive long-term effect. Emerging therapies include endothelin antagonists (bosetan), nitric oxide and phosphodiesterase inhibitors (sildenafil). Lung transplantation may be considered for patients with PH due to parenchymal lung disease or PAV.

Venous thromboembolism and pulmonary embolism

(a) Pulmonary angiograms (A,D) and V/Q scans (B,E = ventilation scans, C,F = perfusion scans) in a normal patient and a patient with a massive right-sided pulmonary embolism. The angiogram (D) shows complete occlusion of the right pulmonary artery. On the V/Q scan there is loss of right lung perfusion (F) but normal ventilation (E)

NORMAL   PULMONARY EMBOLISM

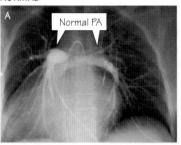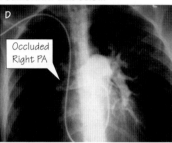

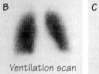 Ventilation scan   Perfusion scan

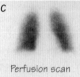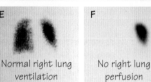 Normal right lung ventilation   No right lung perfusion

(b) Contrast CT scan showing contrast in the heart and pulmonary arteries (PA). Both the right and left PA show irregular defects consistent with pulmonary emboli

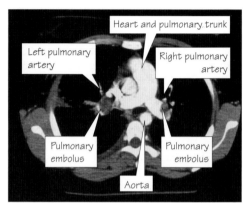

(c) Risk factors for DVT and PE

Surgery	Hip, knee, gynaecological procedures
Trauma	Spinal trauma
General factors	Age, obesity, smoking, oral contraceptive pill (OCP)
Underlying disease	Malignancy, sepsis, stroke, autoimmune disease
Cardiovascular disease	Low flow states (e.g. cardiac failure, immobility) Vascular injury (e.g. atherosclerosis, catheters)
Inherited disorders (less common)	Deficiencies (e.g. antithrombin III, protein C, protein S) Clotting disorders (e.g. Factor V leiden, antiphospholipid syndrome, dysfibrinogenaemias)

(d) DVT prophylaxis

Risk of DVT	Patient	Regime
Low (<1%)	<40 years old, minor surgery (<1h) Minimal immobility	Early ambulation Compression stockings
Moderate (5-10%)	>40 years old, surgery (>1h), cardiac, medical problems, CVA, hypercoagulability	Low dose heparin (UFH or LMWH)
High (>15%)	Complicated surgery, hip or knee surgery, hip fracture, trauma	Full dose LMWH or warfarin

LMWH = low molecular weight heparin
UFH = unfractionated heparin
CVA = cerebrovascular accident

Venous thromboembolism and its most significant complication, **pulmonary embolism (PE)**, are common clinical disorders that have a substantial impact on patient morbidity and mortality; Fig. 27c shows major risks. PE is most often a complication of **deep venous thrombosis (DVT)**. Both disorders are commonly underdiagnosed and require appropriate clinical suspicion and a systematic diagnostic approach. About 5 million patients develop DVT in the USA each year; ~500 000 subsequently develop PE and ~10% of these die. Prophylactic therapy in patients at risk is essential (Fig. 27d); in its absence up to 70% of patients undergoing hip or knee replacement surgery develop DVT.

Deep venous thrombosis

Nearly all clinically significant cases of PE (~90%) arise from DVT in the lower extremities, with thrombi typically originating in the calves and propagating above the knee. Approximately 15–25% will propagate into the femoral and iliac veins and have a 50% risk of embolizing to the lung. Thrombi may develop in the axillary and subclavian veins, usually due to surgery or intravenous catheters, but emboli are usually smaller, with less risk of catastrophic consequences. Soon after thrombus formation, the intrinsic fibrinolytic cascade begins to organize the thrombus. The risk of a thrombus embolizing is greatest early during ongoing proliferation and decreases once it is organized.

Pulmonary embolism

When a thrombus embolizes to the lung, respiratory or circulatory abnormalities occur due to sudden occlusion of a pulmonary artery or arteriole. Occlusion of regional perfusion causes an increase in dead space, necessitating an **increase in minute ventilation** to maintain normal P_aCO_2. Surfactant production distal to the embolus may be reduced after 24 h, resulting in **atelectasis**. **Hypoxaemia** is common and mostly due to V_A/Q **mismatch** (Chapter 14). **Pulmonary infarction** occurs in <25% of cases of PE. Circulatory complications arise from obliteration of the pulmonary vascular bed and a reduction of cardiac output. Severity is related to the amount of lung embolized and the pre-existing state of the pulmonary vasculature and right ventricle (RV). A single large embolus can be catastrophic, whereas multiple small emboli can cause 'pruning' of smaller arteries. Circulatory collapse may occur with >50% obstruction of the pulmonary vascular bed. Less severe emboli may be fatal to patients with pre-existing lung or heart disease.

Clinical features

Clinical features of DVT are non-specific, with lower extremity pain, swelling and erythema. Homan's sign (pain in the calf on dorsiflexion of the foot) occurs in a minority of patients. Fifty per cent of DVTs are undetected.

Most patients with PE have **dyspnoea**, **pleuritic chest pain**, **haemoptysis**, **apprehension** and **tachypnoea**. With severe PE, signs related to **RV failure** (e.g. hypotension, jugular venous distension) may occur. Most patients with PE have non-specific abnormalities on chest X-ray, including atelectasis. The electrocardiogram (ECG) may show non-specific ST segment changes, and rarely, with significant RV strain, an $S_1Q_3T_3$ pattern, right axis deviation (RAD) or right bundle-branch block (RBBB). **Arterial blood gas abnormalities** are common, including **widened A–a gradient**, **hypoxaemia** and **hypocapnia** (despite increased dead space).

Diagnosis

Deep venography or **pulmonary angiography** are the diagnostic standard, although **V/Q scanning** is usually the initial investigation as it is less invasive (Fig. 27a; Chapter 21). A negative perfusion scan effectively rules out PE and a 'high probability' scan (multiple segmental perfusion defects with normal ventilation) has a >85% probability of PE (Fig. 27a). With a high clinical suspicion, a high-probability V/Q scan has a positive predictive value >95%. Unfortunately, most V/Q scans are non-diagnostic or indeterminate, with a 15–50% likelihood of PE, necessitating further imaging. **Non-invasive imaging** of the lower extremity deep veins with Doppler imaging or impedance plethysmography is useful, because the presence of thrombosis requires treatment similar to PE. In patients with underlying cardiac or pulmonary disease, **pulmonary angiography** is indicated if the above tests are not diagnostic. Absence of DVT and a low probability V/Q scan permit treatment to be withheld. **Spiral/helical computed tomography** (CT) has a sensitivity for PE of 70–95% (higher for more proximal emboli) and a specificity >90%. It also allows visualization of parenchymal abnormalities and is in patients with COPD or extensive chest X-ray abnormalities, where V/Q scanning is indeterminate. **Echocardiography** may reveal RV dysfunction in PE and rule out **pericardial tamponade** or severe left ventricular (LV) dysfunction. **Transoesophageal echocardiography** may visualize thromboemboli in the main pulmonary arteries, but not in lobar or segmental arteries.

Treatment

The cornerstone of therapy for DVT/PE is **anticoagulation**, which stops propagation of existing thrombus and allows organization. Immediate therapy in patients with a high suspicion of PE may prevent life-threatening further embolization. **Unfractionated heparin (UFH)** or **low molecular weight heparin (LMWH)** for 5–7 days, followed by **warfarin** for 6 months, is standard therapy. UFH and warfarin must be monitored as subtherapeutic levels increase the risk of recurrent thromboembolism. LMWH is more bioavailable and does not require monitoring. Patients with inherited or acquired hypercoagulability may require lifelong therapy.

In patients with contraindications to anticoagulation (recent surgery, haemorrhagic stroke, central nervous system metastases, active bleeding) or recurrent PE while on therapeutic anticoagulation an **inferior vena cava (IVC) filter** may prevent fatal PE.

Although activation of **fibrinolysis** with **thrombolytics** hastens resolution of perfusion defects and RV dysfunction, convincing benefit is lacking. As thrombolytics cause increased bleeding complications, including a 0.3–1.5% risk of intracerebral haemorrhage, they are only recommended for life-threatening PE with compromised haemodynamics.

(a) CT scan of patient with Wegener's granulomatosis, showing large cavitating masses.

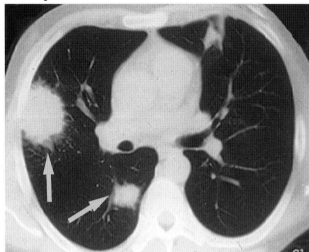

(b) Histological section showing necrobiotic regions with multinucleate giant cells (arrows)

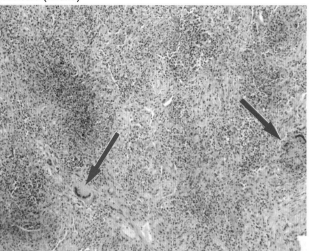

Pulmonary vasculitides.

Disease	Blood vessel	Comment
Collagen vascular diseases		
Rheumatoid arthritis	Arteries/arterioles	Uncommon
Scleroderma	Fibrosis in arterioles	CREST syndrome
SLE	Capillaritis	Pulmonary hemorrhage
Vasculitides		
Wegener's granulomatosis	Granulomatous inflammation	Pulmonary hemorrhage common
	Arteriolar/venular vasculitis	c-ANCA (90%)
	Fibrinoid necrosis	
	Capillaritis (1/3)	
Microscopic polyangiitis	Arteriole/venule vasculitis	Related to Wegener's and PAN
	Capillaritis, fibrinoid necrosis	p-ANCA, hepatitis B, C
Lymphomatoid granulomatosis	Angiocentric/angiodestructive lymphocytes,	Epstein–Barr Virus
	plasma cells, atypical lymphocytes	Lymphoproliferative
Allergic granulomatosis and angiitis	Necrotizing vasculitis in small and	Asthma, eosinophilia
	medium-sized arteries, arterioles, venules	66% p-ANCA or c-ANCA
	Granulomas, eosinophils	
	Fibrinoid necrosis	
Anti-GBM disease	Intra-alveolar haemorrhage	Smoking, recent infection
	Linear IgG in basement membrane	
	Minimal inflammation	

ANCA, antineutrophil cytoplasmic antibody; CREST, calcinosis, Raynaud's phenomenon, esophageal involvement, sclerodactyly and telangiectasia; GBM, glomerular basement membrane; PAN, polyarteritis nodosa; SLE, systemic lupus erythematosus.

Immunologically mediated **vascular inflammation** is common to the various types of **systemic vasculitis**. Vasculitis may be secondary to systemic **collagen vascular disease**—such as **rheumatoid arthritis, scleroderma** or **systemic lupus erythematosus (SLE)**—or may be **primary vasculitides** that involve pulmonary blood vessels (**Wegener's granulomatosis, microscopic polyangiitis, lymphomatoid granulomatosis, allergic granulomatosis** and **angiitis**). Antiglomerular basement membrane disease (**Goodpasture's syndrome**) has a similar clinical presentation to pulmonary vasculitis. Most of these disorders show systemic symptoms including a **characteristic rash**, and may cause pulmonary infiltrates, masses, necrotizing lesions or alveolar haemorrhage.

Systemic vasculitis is commonly associated with the presence of autoantibodies against components of the cytoplasm of normal granulocytes and neutrophils. **Antineutrophil cytoplasmic antibodies (ANCA)** can be used as diagnostic markers; the two forms are peroxidase-1 **PR3-ANCA** and myeloperoxidase **MPO-ANCA** (old names c-ANCA and p-ANCA).

Collagen vascular diseases

Rheumatoid arthritis may cause vasculitis and **pulmonary hypertension** (Chapter 26); however, this is far less frequent than pleural disease (Chapter 30) or diffuse parenchymal disease (Chapter 29). Patients may develop **Caplan's syndrome** as a result of dust inhalation (e.g. coal dust) (Chapter 31). **Limited cutaneous scleroderma** often spares lung parenchyma and causes pulmonary hypertension by direct involvement of pulmonary arterioles. While not common, **pulmonary capillaritis** causing alveolar haemorrhage secondary to **SLE** is a devastating complication with a high mortality rate. Patients generally have a pre-existing diagnosis of SLE, usually with renal involvement. Rarely, SLE may cause pulmonary hypertension by direct involvement of the pulmonary vasculature. Clinically, this is indistinguishable from **pulmonary arterial hypertension** (Chapter 26).

Granulomatoses

Wegener's granulomatosis (WG) is a systemic vasculitis that predominantly involves the upper and lower respiratory systems and the renal glomeruli. Vascular inflammation may involve arterioles, capillaries and venules. Patients are generally aged 40–60 years and present with upper respiratory symptoms usually involving the sinuses (sinusitis) or nasopharynx (ulcers, septal perforation, saddle nose deformity). Radiographic abnormalities in the chest are common, mostly as nodules or masses, often with cavitation (Fig. 28a), but they may appear as parenchymal infiltrates. Renal disease is usual and consists of glomerulonephritis with haematuria, proteinuria and red blood cell casts. Necrotizing **granulomas** (chronically inflamed tissue masses characterized by multinucleate giant cells) are seen in the lungs (Fig. 28b), nasopharynx and kidneys. WG may also involve the ears (otitis media), eyes (conjunctivitis, uveitis), heart (coronary arteries), peripheral nervous system, skin or joints. PR3-ANCA has a 60–90% sensitivity and >90% specificity for WG.

Microscopic polyangiitis has microscopic similarities to WG and polyarteritis nodosa. In contrast to WG, MPA does not involve the nasopharynx and sinuses and is usually associated with MPO-ANCA rather PR3-ANCA. It is often seen in patients with hepatitis B or C

infection. **Treatment** with corticosteroids and cyclophosphamide substantially reduces mortality.

Lymphomatoid granulomatosis (LG) is a systemic vasculitis of lungs, kidneys, central nervous system (CNS) and skin. LG is strongly associated with, and may be a late complication of, **Epstein–Barr virus** (EBV) infection. It behaves like an indolent lymphoproliferative disease and may transform into a B-cell lymphoma. Patients typically have fever, malaise, cough, dyspnoea and a papular rash. Radiographic abnormalities usually consist of multiple lower lobe nodular densities. Lung biopsy shows angiocentric/angiodestructive mixed cell infiltration with lymphocytes, plasma cells and atypical lymphocytes. Vascular occlusion and necrosis are common. **Treatment:** LG is considered to be a lymphoproliferative disorder and is treated with chemotherapy and corticosteroids. Without treatment, the disease progresses and is usually fatal.

Allergic granulomatosis and angiitis (*Churg–Strauss syndrome*) is a medium/small vessel granulomatous vasculitis of the lung, skin, heart, nervous system and kidney. It is probably the second most common pulmonary vasculitis after WG. Most patients have a history of allergic rhinitis and/or asthma and peripheral eosinophilia that may predate the vasculitis by up to a decade. Patients will present with worsening asthma, fever, malaise, subcutaneous tender nodules, mononeuritis multiplex and radiographic infiltrates. There may also be pericarditis, abdominal pain and glomerulonephritis. Radiographic abnormalities are most often patchy, fleeting infiltrates, but may include cavitating nodules or masses, interstitial infiltrates or pleural effusions. CT scans may show ground glass opacities or peribronchial thickening. Lung biopsy shows perivascular granulomatous inflammation, small artery and vein vasculitis, prominent eosinophils and necrosis. The diagnosis may be made without biopsy in the presence of asthma, eosinophilia, migratory pulmonary infiltrates and neuropathy. Both PR3-ANCA and MPO-ANCA may be positive. **Treatment:** most patients respond to corticosteroids. Cyclophosphamide or azathioprine may be added in resistant cases. Patients who respond to therapy seldom relapse. Patients with an onset of asthma immediately before or concurrent with vasculitis have a poorer prognosis. Overall, survival is >70%, with mortality due to cardiac, CNS, renal or gastrointestinal involvement.

Anti-glomerular basement membrane (GBM) disease is caused by antibodies directed against the glomerular membranes causing glomerulonephritis. In **Goodpasture's syndrome** these antibodies sometimes cross-react with alveolar basement membrane, causing alveolar haemorrhage. Alveolar haemorrhage occurs predominantly in smokers, or after recent respiratory infections that alter alveolar permeability. Patients present with rapidly progressive glomerulonephritis, haemoptysis, anaemia and diffuse alveolar infiltrates on radiographs. In contrast to the primary vasculitides, prolonged systemic symptoms are uncommon. Pulmonary function testing demonstrates elevated $D_{L}CO$ from extravasated haemoglobin in the lung. Diagnosis requires demonstration of anti-GBM antibodies in serum or linear IgG in glomerular or alveolar basement membranes. Both PR3-ANCA and MPO-ANCA may be positive. **Treatment:** patients with Goodpasture's syndrome should be treated with plasmapheresis, cyclophosphamide and corticosteroids. Therapy may control alveolar haemorrhage; however, renal disease is usually irreversible if the presenting creatinine is >5 mg/dL.

Interstitial lung disease

(a) The interstitium of the lung and cellular basis of fibrosis (not to scale)

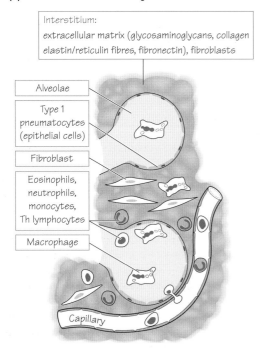

Interstitium:
extracellular matrix (glycosaminoglycans, collagen
elastin/reticulin fibres, fibronectin), fibroblasts

Alveolae

Type 1
pneumatocytes
(epithelial cells)

Fibroblast

Eosinophils,
neutrophils,
monocytes,
Th lymphocytes

Macrophage

Capillary

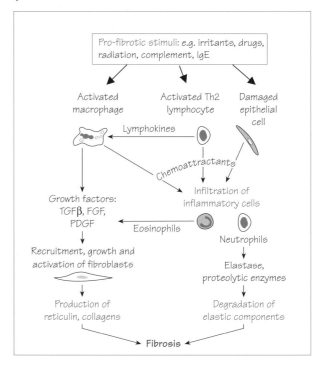

Pro-fibrotic stimuli: e.g. irritants, drugs,
radiation, complement, IgE

Activated
macrophage → Lymphokines ← Activated Th2
lymphocyte

Damaged
epithelial
cell

Chemoattractants

Growth factors:
TGFβ, FGF,
PDGF ← Eosinophils

Infiltration of
inflammatory cells

Neutrophils

Recruitment, growth and
activation of fibroblasts

Elastase,
proteolytic enzymes

Production of
reticulin, collagens

Degradation of
elastic components

Fibrosis

Initial stimuli (e.g. irritants, pollutants, autoimmune) activate macrophages and Th lymphocytes and/or damage epithelial cells
leading to an inflammatory response, production of growth factors and fibrosis. (Diagram highly simplified)
Key growth factors: TGFβ (transforming growth factor), FGF (fibroblast growth factor), PDGF (platelet-derived growth factor).

(b) High resolution CT scan showing ground glass shadowing and mosaic pattern typical of alveolitis (1), and normal region (2)

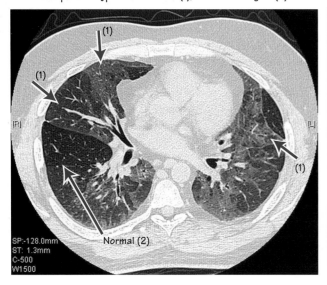

(1)

(1)

(1)

Normal (2)

SP:-128.0mm
ST: 1.3mm
C-500
W1500

(c) CT of patient with cryptogenic fibrosing alveolitis and UIP Note peripheral distribution of fibrotic change (3)

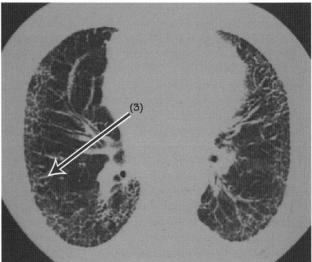

(3)

Interstitial lung disease refers to an extensive variety of acute and chronic disorders, characterized by **inflammation** or **fibrosis** of alveolar–capillary units and distal airways (Fig. 29a). As these diseases are not limited to the interstitium but may involve matrix components throughout the lung, a more accurate description is *'diffuse parenchymal lung disease'*. Causes include **respiratory diseases** (e.g. pneumonias, sarcoidosis), **autoimmune diseases, drugs and therapies** (e.g. bleomycin, oxygen, radiation) and **occupational/environmental factors** (Chapter 31).

Clinical features

Dyspnoea and **cough** are common, usually indolent over months, with **digital clubbing** and **diffuse inspiratory crackles**. **Hypoxaemia** and right ventricular failure may develop in advanced disease. Pulmonary function tests (Chapter 20) reveal reduced **total lung capacity** (TLC), **functional residual capacity** (FRC) and **residual volume** (RV) due to **decreased compliance** and **increased elastic recoil** of the lungs. $D_L CO$ is deceased due to diminished surface area for gas exchange secondary to reduced lung volume. Exercise induces rapid shallow breathing and O_2 desaturation.

Most (>90%) interstitial lung disease patients have an **abnormal chest X-ray (CXR)**, with any combination of alveolar, interstitial or mixed infiltrates, typically predominating in the lower lobes. Small (0.5–2 cm), thick-walled cysts denote advanced fibrosis and give rise to a typical radiological appearance known as **'honeycomb lung'**. High-resolution computed tomography (HRCT) allows a far more accurate distinction of parenchymal involvement. **Bronchoalveolar lavage (BAL)** may be useful to diagnose malignancy, eosinophilic pneumonia, alveolar proteinosis or alveolar haemorrhage. BAL fluid containing increased inflammatory cells (Chapter 18) reflects alveolitis and correlates with ground glass infiltrates on HRCT (Fig. 29b); this may identify patients with rapidly progressive or potentially reversible disease. **Open** or **thoracoscopic lung biopsy** is usually necessary to determine a diagnosis and therapeutic plan.

Classification may be clinical or histological. Clinically, interstitial lung disease may be caused by occupational or environmental exposures (Chapter 31), drugs/therapies, autoimmune diseases and primary pulmonary conditions or may be idiopathic. Histological patterns include usual interstitial pneumonia (**UIP**), desquamative interstitial pneumonia (**DIP**), non-specific interstitial pneumonia (**NSIP**), acute interstitial pneumonitis (**AIP**, *Hamman–Rich syndrome*), lymphocytic interstitial pneumonia (**LIP**), organizing pneumonia, eosinophilic pneumonia, granulomatous disease or honeycomb lung. Histological patterns are usually not disease-specific.

Idiopathic pulmonary fibrosis/cryptogenic fibrosing alveolitis

This typically occurs in men in their 60s, with lower lobe subpleural fibrosis. The most common histological pattern is UIP, although this may represent a point in progression of DIP or NSIP to end-stage honeycomb lung. UIP is a patchy disease with areas of normal lung, interstitial inflammation and fibrosis with fibroblast proliferation (Figs 29a and c). UIP can be reliably diagnosed on CT scan, based on peripheral distribution (Fig. 29c). Median survival with UIP is <5 years; *corticosteroids have minimal effect.* DIP and NSIP are diagnosed at younger ages, have more diffuse, more cellular, less fibrotic involvement and *respond well to corticosteroids.* Mean survival with DIP and NSIP is >10 years; complete recovery is attainable. These differences highlight the utility of histological examination.

Sarcoidosis

This is a multiorgan granulomatous disease of unknown aetiology, but with characteristic clinical and pathological features. Activated CD4 lymphocytes appear to participate in the pathophysiology. Sarcoidosis is usually asymptomatic, presenting with unsuspected bilateral hilar adenopathy on CXR in the young (20–40 years). Symptomatic sarcoidosis most often involves the lung, but may also be present in eyes, skin, joints, central nervous system (CNS), heart or liver. Radiographically, lung disease manifests as any combination of **hilar/paratracheal adenopathy, reticulonodular infiltrates** or **advanced fibrosis with cysts**. Nevertheless, physical examination may be normal. Pleural disease is uncommon. **Non-caseating granulomas** are a classic histological feature of sarcoidosis. **Angiotensin-converting enzyme** is commonly elevated.

Sarcoidosis is usually **self-limiting without therapy**—up to 50% of cases resolve without treatment within 3 years. However, some patients develop progressive interstitial lung disease involvement and should be followed with periodic radiographs and pulmonary function tests. Therapy is indicated for significant organ involvement or impairment on pulmonary function testing. Oral **corticosteroids** are standard therapy and most patients achieve remission within months; optimal duration of therapy is variable. Immunomodulation or suppression may benefit selected patients but no benefit over corticosteroids has been shown. Lung transplantation is an option for patients with advanced fibrosis.

Autoimmune and collagen vascular disease

Interstitial lung disease is a common complication of such disorders, but must be distinguished from complications due to drug therapy or opportunistic infections. Patients have signs, symptoms, CXR and pulmonary function tests similar to those with idiopathic pulmonary fibrosis or AIP. Symptomatic disease may respond to aggressive therapy with chemotherapeutic agents plus corticosteroids.

Scleroderma: up to 70% of patients may have interstitial fibrosis. A ground-glass pattern on HRCT or alveolitis on BAL is associated with more rapid deterioration of lung function. Median survival is 8 years.

Rheumatoid arthritis: interstitial lung disease is common, with males, smokers and patients with severe joint disease at highest risk.

Polymyositis/dermatomyositis: a rare disorder of unknown cause, possibly autoimmune, dominated by slowly progressing inflammation of striated muscle. Fifty per cent of patients develop interstitial lung disease, a frequent cause of mortality.

Systemic lupus erythematosus (SLE) has a <10% incidence of acute and chronic interstitial pneumonitis, whereas in **Sjögren's syndrome** the most common interstitial lung disease is LIP, which may evolve to **pulmonary lymphoma**.

30 Pleural diseases

(a) Causes of pleural effusions

EXUDATIVE:
(protein ratio pleural/serum >0.5 OR LDH ratio pleural/serum >0.6 OR pleural LDH > 0.66 of top normal serum value)

Infectious

Para-pneumonic
- aerobic bacterial pneumonia
- anaerobic bacterial pneumonia

Empyema

Tuberculosis

Parasitic
- amoeba
- echinococcus
- paragonimus

Viral

Autoimmune/collagen vascular

Systemic lupus erythematosus

Rheumatoid arthritis

Neoplastic

Lung cancer

Metastatic disease

Mesothelioma

Abdominal

Pancreatitis/pseudocyst

Oesophageal rupture

Liver abscess

Splenic abscess

Miscellaneous

Pulmonary embolism

Drug reactions

Asbestos exposure

Haemothorax

Chylothorax

Post-cardiac surgery

Post-myocardial infarction

Meig's syndrome

TRANSUDATIVE:
(meets NONE of the criteria for exudative)

Congestive heart failure

Cirrhosis
Hepatic hydrothorax

Myxoedema

Nephrotic disease

Peritoneal dialysis

(b) CXR showing large pleural effusion in left lung (contrast with pneumothorax CXR in Chapter 33)

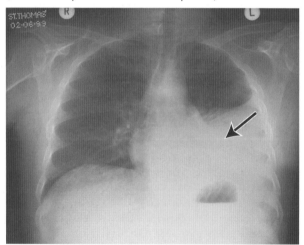

(c) CT scan demonstrating irregular (lumpy) pleural thickening of mesothelioma over lateral right chest wall (see arrows)

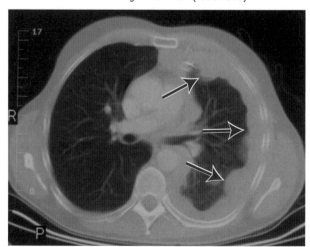

The pleurae

The potential space between the **parietal** and **visceral pleurae** serves as a coupling system between the lung and the chest wall, and normally contains a small amount of fluid. A negative pleural pressure is maintained by the dynamic tension between the chest wall and the lung (Chapter 3). Both pleurae have a systemic blood supply and lymphatics, although lymphatic drainage of the pleural space is predominantly via the parietal pleura. Fluid flux through the pleural space is determined by Starling's relationship between microvascular pressures, oncotic pressures, permeability and surface area. Normally, there is net filtration of **transudative** (protein-poor) fluid into the pleural space that is balanced by resorption via the parietal lymphatics.

Pneumothorax is an important condition that occurs when air enters the pleural space and pleural pressure rises to atmospheric pressure; pneumothorax is discussed in detail in Chapter 33.

Chylothorax is due to accumulation of triglyceride-rich lymph in the pleural space, generally as the result of damage to the thoracic duct causing leakage into the pleural space, for example due to trauma or carcinoma.

Empyema is accumulation of pus.

Pleurisy is a term commonly used to describe the sharp localized pain arising from any disease of the pleura. It is made worse by deep inspiration and coughing.

Pathophysiology

Most diseases of the pleura present with **pleural effusion**, which can be detected on chest X-ray (CXR) when >300 mL of fluid is present (Fig. 30b). Effusions are due to excessive fluid formation or inadequate fluid clearance. Symptoms develop if the fluid is **inflammatory** or if **pulmonary mechanics** are compromised. Thus, the most common symptoms of a pleural effusion are **pleuritic chest pain**, **dull aching pain**, **fullness of the chest** or **dyspnoea**. Physical examination reveals decreased breath sounds, dullness to percussion, decreased tactile or vocal fremitus. If there is inflammation, there may be a friction rub. **Compressive atelectasis** (partial lung collapse) may cause bronchial breath sounds.

It is useful to categorize pleural effusions as **transudative** or **exudative** (Fig. 30a).

Transudative effusions are usually due to an imbalance in Starling's forces across normal pleural membranes, have protein-poor fluid, are often bilateral and are not associated with fever, pleuritic pain or tenderness to palpation. The most common cause of a transudative effusion is **congestive heart failure**. Other causes include cirrhosis with ascites, nephrotic syndrome, pericardial disease or peritoneal dialysis.

Exudative effusions imply disease of the pleura or the adjacent lung and are characterized by an increased protein, lactate dehydrogenase (LDH), cholesterol or white blood cell count (WBC) (Fig. 30a). The differential diagnosis of exudative effusions is broad, including infection, malignancy, autoimmune disease, oesophageal perforation and pancreatitis.

Diagnostic evaluation of pleural effusion should include measurement of pleural aspirate cell count with differential, pH, protein, LDH, cholesterol and glucose. These studies usually distinguish exudates from transudates and will often suggest a specific diagnosis. For example, extremely low glucose is typical for empyema, malignancy, tuberculosis (Chapter 36), rheumatoid arthritis, systemic lupus erythematosus (SLE) or oesophageal perforation. If clinically indicated, a specific diagnosis may be obtained from microbiological stains and culture, cytopathology, amylase, triglycerides and measurement of antinuclear antibody (ANA) titre. Although all patients with SLE have a positive ANA titre in the pleural fluid, it is also present in a significant proportion (~15%) of other effusions; these may be related to malignancy.

Treatment is for the underlying condition, but persistent or reaccumulating effusions can be drained to dryness (slowly so as to avoid severe pain).

Specific conditions

Pneumonia (Chapters 34 & 35) commonly causes parapneumonic pleural effusions. These effusions are usually sterile exudates with a neutrophilic leukocytosis and require only treatment of the pneumonia to resolve. However, if bacteria invade the pleural space, a complicated parapneumonic effusion or empyema will develop. These effusions are characterized by a low pH and extensive fibrin deposition causing fluid loculation and require adequate open or closed drainage for healing. *Streptococcus pneumoniae*, *Staphylococcus aureus*, Gram-negative bacteria and anaerobes commonly cause complicated effusions.

Tuberculosis pleurisy occurs when a subpleural focus of primary infection ruptures into the pleural space, causing a delayed hypersensitivity response. Subsequently, an exudative effusion with a lymphocytic leukocytosis, a paucity of macrophages and an elevated adenosine deaminase will develop. Patients develop fever, dyspnoea, pleuritic pain and a positive tuberculin response (Chapter 36). Granulomatous inflammation is seen on pleural biopsy and culture of pleural tissue has the highest diagnostic yield.

Primary lung malignancies or **metastases** to the lung may cause pleural effusions by direct invasion or by obstruction of parietal lymphatic drainage. Malignant effusions are mostly exudative (90%), often with a very high LDH, low pH and low glucose. Cytology of the pleural fluid has a high diagnostic yield. Symptomatic pleural effusions may respond to therapy for the underlying malignancy, although palliative obliteration of the pleural space (**pleurodesis**) is often necessary to relieve dyspnoea or chest pain.

Mesothelioma is an uncommon malignancy that originates in the pleura and/or peritoneum (Chapter 31). Over 75% of cases develop 20–30 years after occupational asbestos exposure. Asbestos may also cause benign pleural effusions or calcified plaques on the parietal pleura in the lower lungs or along the diaphragmatic surface. Mesothelioma typically develops in men aged 50–70 years, presenting with insidious dyspnoea and aching chest pain. Chest X-rays usually show unilateral pleural effusion (Fig. 30b), and computed tomography (CT) shows lumpy fibrotic encasement of the pleural space (Fig. 30c). Pleural fluid cytology is not usually diagnostic. Thoracoscopic biopsies have the highest yield. Treatment is generally palliative, including pleurodesis. The prognosis is poor, with a median survival of approximately 1 year.

31 Occupational and environmental-related lung disease

(a) Common examples of irritant gases and other agents causing lung-specific responses

Agent	Source	Response
Ammonia	Industrial refrigeration leaks, fertilizers	**Low exposure** Exacerbations of asthma and COPD Enhanced response to allergen
Chlorine gas	Industrial leakage, water purification including swimming pools, household bleach (liquid/powder) interactions	**Moderate exposure** Mild mucosal irritation Airway inflammation and bronchiolitis
Hydrogen sulphide	Sewers and manure pits, fossil fuel extraction	**Severe exposure** Epithelial damage leading to diffuse alveolar damage Pulmonary oedema and ARDS
Nitrogen dioxide Nitrogen oxides	Vehicle exhausts, welding, power stations, oil refineries, gas and oil burning equipment, organic decomposition, structural or polymer fibres	**In some cases – late response (2–8 weeks)** Bronchiolitis obliterans after initial recovery
Ozone	Vehicle exhausts, welding, copiers, ozone generators, bleaching, water treatment, plasma welding	
Sulphur dioxide	Combustion of fossil fuels, power stations, oil refineries, smelters, oil burning heaters, mining, ore refining, cement manufacturing, refrigeration plants	**Also:** direct bronchoconstriction, especially in asthmatics
Acrolein, aldehydes	Structural or wildland fires, other combustion	**Also:** strongly pro-inflammatory (esp. acrolein)
Diesel particulates (<10 μm)	Diesel engines	Airway/alveolar inflammation Increased deaths in elderly
Heavy metals (cadmium, mercury)	Welding, brazing, metal cutting, metal reclamation	Acute pneumonitis 12–24 hours after exposure
Paraquat	Ingestion of herbicides	Accelerated, chemically induced pulmonary fibrosis
Polycyclic hydrocarbons Hydrocarbons	Diesel exhaust, tobacco smoke Ingestion of hydrocarbons (children)	Cancer Aspiration hydrocarbon pneumonitis

(b) Typical causes of allergic alveolitis

Disease/occupation	Material	Causative agent
Farmer's lung	Mouldy hay or other vegetable matter	Thermophilic actinomycetes bacteria (Saccharopolyspora rectivirgula, Thermoactinomyces species)
Bagassosis	Sugar cane	
Mushroom workers	Compost	
Humidifier fever	Contaminated water	– Also Klebsiella oxytoca, amoebae
Pigeon fancier's (breeder's) lung	Feathers and excreta	Avian proteins
Farmers, sawmill, tobacco, esparto grass and brewery workers	Fungal contamination of materials	Primarily Aspergillus species
Cheese, laboratory, cork workers	Fungal contamination of materials	Primarily Penicillium species
Household	Fungal infestations of damp walls and woodwork	Multiple fungal species
– other bacterial causes	Contamination of water, wood shavings, etc	Bacillus subtilis, Klebsiella, Epicoccum nigrum, non-tubercular mycobacteria

The most common form of occupational and environmental lung disease is **asthma** (Chapters 23 & 24). The UK government has reported that 750 000 people with asthma work in an environment that triggers their symptoms, and >3000 per year develop asthma as a result of workplace substances. While the most common cause of occupational asthma is isocyanates (e.g. paint and plastics), grain and flour dust are not far behind, and secondary smoking is most commonly reported to exacerbate symptoms. It is estimated that elimination of occupational asthma alone could have a benefit of up to £1 billion over 10 years; education and prevention are therefore key targets.

Response to acute lung irritants

Inhaled irritants (Fig. 31a) cause exacerbation of asthma and chronic obstructive pulmonary disease (COPD), coughing and dyspnoea through activation of irritant receptors (Chapter 12), and irritation of mucus membranes. Highly soluble agents (e.g. ammonia, sulphur dioxide) cause immediate irritation in the upper airways, whereas less soluble agents (e.g. chlorine, ozone) favour deeper penetration to alveolar epithelial cells, which are particularly susceptible to injury. High concentrations lead to extensive lung injury, primarily by damage to epithelium, consequent inflammation and **pulmonary oedema**. Development of **acute respiratory distress syndrome** (ARDS) is common, and treatment is similar (Chapter 40). Some patients who initially recover from moderate or severe exposure may subsequently develop **bronchiolitis obliterans** (obliteration of bronchioles by fibrous growth) after 2–8 weeks. Although steroids may slow progression, prognosis is often poor.

Inhalation of mineral dusts (pneumoconiosis)

Coal worker's pneumoconiosis (CWP) is caused by inhalation of coal or carbon dust. In **simple CWP**, the upper lobes of the lung contain small (<4 mm), round opacities (coal macules) consisting of dust, dust-laden macrophages and fibroblasts. These may enlarge to fibrosed coal nodules. Weakening of bronchiolar walls leads to focal emphysema, which together with macules is characteristic of CWP. Simple CWP is often described as symptomless, with no change in lung function. It can, however, develop into **progressive massive fibrosis** (PMF), with black fibrotic masses from 1 cm to several centimeters in diameter, which may have necrotic cavities. Obliteration and disruption of airways results in emphysema. Patients show irreversible airflow limitation, loss of lung volume and elastic recoil, and reduced $D_{L}CO$, with breathlessness on exertion. Treatment is limited, and similar to other progressive fibrotic diseases (Chapter 24). **Caplan's syndrome** is a nodular form of CWP associated with the defective immunology of rheumatoid disease; it may also occur with asbestosis or silicosis.

Asbestos is a fibrous mixture of silicates that is highly resistant to degradation. The fibres are 1–2 μm wide, but up to 50 μm (**blue asbestos**; crocidolite) or 2 cm (**white asbestos**; chrysotile) long. They are thus easily trapped in the lung. Blue asbestos is far more dangerous. Regulations have reduced exposure since the 1980s, but the presence of asbestos in buildings and the long interval between exposure and disease development mean that asbestos-related disease will be encountered for some time. **Asbestos bodies** (protein-covered fibres)

in the lungs are indicative of exposure, but not disease. The type and extent of disease largely depend on exposure. **Asbestosis** is a fibrous lung disease developing up to 10 years after heavy exposure. Patients present with progressive dyspnoea, basal crackles on inspiration and sometimes finger clubbing. There is a restrictive lung function defect and reduced $D_{L}CO$, with diffuse streaky shadows on X-ray and thickening of visceral pleura; **honeycomb lung** is often prominent in the lower lobes. Prognosis is poor. **Mesothelioma** (Chapter 30) can develop up to 40 years after light exposure, and is invariably fatal. Milder forms of asbestos-induced pleural disease produce dyspnoea and restrictive defects coupled with pleural thickening and plaques or effusions, with scattered fibrotic foci. No treatment is effective for asbestos-related disease, as the stimulus remains in the lungs. Asbestos-related lung cancer is discussed in Chapter 39.

Silicosis is a fibrotic disease caused by inhalation of silica, with a low prevalence in developed nations. Occupations at risk include mining, stoneworking, manufacture of abrasives, foundry work and glassworking. Silica is very toxic to macrophages and thus highly fibrogenic. Chronic silicosis (over decades) is characterized by **silicotic nodules** of collagen around a cell-free core, first developing in hilar lymph nodes. In acute silicosis due to heavy exposure, severe dyspnoea may develop over months. The clinical features of silicosis are similar to PMF.

Inhalation of organic material

Extrinsic allergic alveolitis (or **hypersensitivity pneumonitis**) is a diffuse inflammatory disease of small airways and alveoli caused by allergens, primarily microbial spores, that are small enough to reach the alveoli (Fig. 31b). The most common example is **farmer's lung**, caused by dust from mouldy hay or plants contaminated with **thermophilic actinomycetes** bacteria, which thrive in warm moist conditions. Typically, symptoms occur several hours after exposure, and include fever, dyspnoea and cough. Although early removal of exposure results in rapid recovery, continuous exposure leads to progressive **interstitial fibrosis** (Chapter 30), with infiltration of inflammatory cells and formation of **granulomas** (chronically inflamed tissue masses characterized by multinucleate giant cells, see Fig. 28b). Patients present with dyspnoea, restrictive defects and decreased $D_{L}CO$. Fluffy nodular shadowing or ground glass opacity may be shown in CXR, with honeycomb lung (Chapter 30) in severe cases. Detailed histories are required to establish antigens, with confirmation by precipitating antibodies in serum. **Management** centres on abolishing antigen exposure. High-dose corticosteroids can regress early disease, but established disease with fibrosis is irreversible and can progress to respiratory failure. **Differential diagnosis** includes asthma (Chapters 23 & 24), sarcoidosis (Chapter 29), viral and mycoplasma pneumonias (Chapters 34 & 35) and mycobacterial infections.

Byssinosis occurs in workers handling raw cotton, flax and hemp. It is characterized by chest tightness, cough and/or shortness of breath on the first day back at work, with recovery as the week progresses. It is primarily due to acute bronchoconstriction, possibly related to contaminating bacterial endotoxins. Long-term exposure causes a disease similar to chronic bronchitis (Chapter 25), with chronic productive cough, progressive decline in lung function and disability.

(a) Mean survival of CF patients

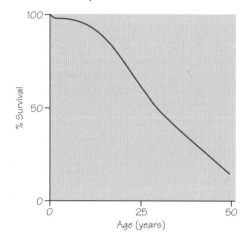

(b) Development of respiratory problems in CF

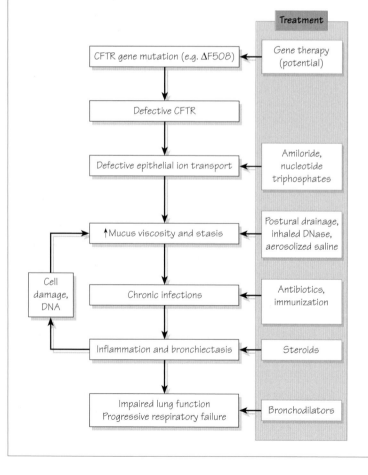

(c) Other conditions associated with CF

Condition	% of CF patents
Delayed development, puberty	100%
Male infertility (absent/obstructed vas deferens and epididymis)	98%
Female infertility	20%
Pancreatic insufficiency	85%
Nasal polyps	15–20%, most in 2nd decade
Symptomatic sinusitis	10% children 25% adults
Rectal prolapse	20% children Rare in adults
Bone demineralization (vitamin D deficiency)	Common
Hypertrophic osteoarthropathy	15% adults
Dysfunctional gallbladder or gallstones	10–30%
Biliary cirrhosis	5% adults

(d) Some conditions associated with bronchiectasi

Allergic bronchopulmonary aspergillosis (Chapter 31)
α_1-antitrypsin deficiency (Chapters 18, 25)
Bronchial obstruction (foreign bodies, mucus, tumour)
Congenital cartilage deficiency (Williams–Campbell syndrome)
Cystic fibrosis
Fibrotic disease and alveolitis (Chapters 29, 31)
HIV and immunodeficiency (Chapter 37)
Infection (e.g. measles, pertussis), pneumonia (Chapters 34, 35)
Lung transplant
Primary ciliary dyskinesia (Kartagener's syndrome, Chapter 18)
Rheumatoid arthritis
Tuberculosis (Chapter 36)
Tracheobronchomegaly (Mounier–Kuhn syndrome)

Cystic fibrosis (CF) is the primary cause of severe chronic lung disease in children, although 90% of children now survive into their second decade (Fig. 32a). CF is characterized by **chronic bronchopulmonary infection** and airway obstruction (Fig. 32b) and by **exocrine pancreatic insufficiency** with consequent effects on gut function, nutrition and development. The key feature of CF is **increased viscosity** and **subsequent stasis of epithelial mucus**. There is usually an **increased salt content of sweat**. Figure 32c shows some associated disorders.

CF is an **autosomal recessive trait** that is the most common genetic cause of morbidity and mortality in the white population, with a prevalence of approximately one in 2000 live births; nearly 5% of white people of European descent are heterozygous carriers. Prevalence is far less in others, being ~1 in 17 000 for those of African descent. CF is due to mutations in a gene on chromosome 7 encoding for the **cystic fibrosis transmembrane conductance regulator** (CFTR), a cyclic adenosine monophosphate (cAMP)-regulated epithelial chloride channel that can also alter activity of other ionic transporters. Dysfunction of CFTR impairs epithelial chloride, sodium and water transfer and thus causes **reduced mucus hydration** and **increased viscosity** (Chapter 18). Over 800 mutations in the CFTR gene have been described, but the most common, found in ~65% of patients with CF, is deletion of the phenylalanine codon at position 508, the **ΔF508** mutation.

Clinical features

The lungs of neonates with CF are often normal, but rapid development of respiratory symptoms, including refractory cough and infections, is usual. CF patients nearly always have an increased lung volume and **finger clubbing** (increased curvature of the nail and loss of normal angle between nail and nail bed) (Chapter 19). Recurrent bronchopulmonary infections, primarily as a result of defective mucus clearance, are rarely cleared once established and eventually result in **bronchiectasis** (see below), extensive lung damage and dysfunction. Spontaneous **pneumothorax** (Chapter 33) and **haemoptysis** (spitting blood; Chapter 44) are not uncommon. About 10% of neonates present with meconium ileus (failure to pass meconium), which can cause death in the first days of life; 20% of older patients exhibit a similar ileal obstruction (**meconium ileus equivalent**, MIE). Eighty-five per cent of patients have steatorrhoea (high fat stools) as a result of pancreatic insufficiency. Some patients have only mild respiratory symptoms for many years, but this is inevitably followed by a characteristic increase in the frequency and severity of periods of exacerbation of symptoms (cough, dyspnoea, loss of appetite). Eventually, severe restrictions in activity herald the end-stage disease, followed by respiratory failure, hypoxaemia, pulmonary hypertension and death.

Diagnosis

Several factors need to be taken into account, including a **family history** of the disease and the presence of typical respiratory and gastrointestinal disorders (Fig. 32c). A **sweat chloride or sodium** concentration above 60 mmol/L is diagnostic when coupled with such disorders, although ~1% of CF patients may have normal sweat electrolytes. DNA analysis can detect known mutations (e.g. ΔF508), but is limited by the high number of unknown mutations. In later disease, chest X-rays can detect bronchiectasis (see below). Neonates can be screened for CF by blood immunoreactive trypsin, which can detect many, but not all cases.

Management

The primary objectives of treatment are to **control infection, promote mucus clearance** and **improve nutrition**. Early antibiotic therapy is crucial to inhibit progression of the disease. Choice of antibiotic is determined following identification of infecting organisms. The dosage should be higher in CF patients and the course longer. Development of resistance is a key problem and is transferable; segregation of patients is thus advisable. Adequate immunization for measles, pertussis and influenza is important, as these organisms are particularly dangerous in CF.

Clearance: training by physiotherapists in postural drainage (tipping the body so that the infected lobe is uppermost) is vital, coupled with chest percussion to mobilize secretions to the upper airways where they can be coughed up. Such treatment is prescribed one to four times a day. Recently introduced therapies include inhalation of DNase, an enzyme that breaks down DNA from dead cells, which contributes to mucus viscosity. Inhalation of aerosolized saline may improve mucus hydration, as may blockade of sodium reabsorption with amiloride or stimulation of chloride secretion with nucleotide triphosphates. Cough should never be suppressed, as it is an important method of clearance.

Other therapies: bronchodilators (β-agonists) may improve lung function and corticosteroids may assist inflammation in some patients. A potential therapy under intense investigation is gene transfer of the normal CFTR gene. In end-stage respiratory disease a lung transplant should be considered.

Nutrition: most patients with CF require pancreatic enzymes with meals, supplemented with vitamins. High-calorific foods should be advised.

Bronchiectasis

Bronchiectasis is an abnormal and permanent dilatation of proximal (>2 mm) bronchi due to inflammation and subsequent destruction of the elastic and muscular components of their walls (Chapter 44). It is normally associated with defects in **mucociliary clearance** (Chapter 18) and **persistent respiratory infections**. Onset is often in childhood, following pulmonary infections complicating measles or pertussis. Since the introduction of antibiotics, the most common cause of bronchiectasis is now CF (Fig. 32d), except in poorly resourced countries. Symptoms depend on the severity and location of diseased bronchi, but commonly include persistent productive cough, with large quantities of foul-smelling purulent sputum as the disease worsens. Severity has been correlated with the volume of sputum produced, but not with dyspnoea. Haemoptysis and recurrent pneumonia or abscesses are common; haemoptysis is normally mild, but can become life-threatening, particularly in CF patients. Fever, anaemia and weight loss may accompany the disease. Patients often develop finger clubbing, metastatic abscesses, respiratory failure and amyloidosis. Chest X-rays and high-resolution computed tomography (HRCT) can often detect the dilated and thickened bronchi (Chapter 44). **Management** is similar to that for CF, although without the nutritional requirements.

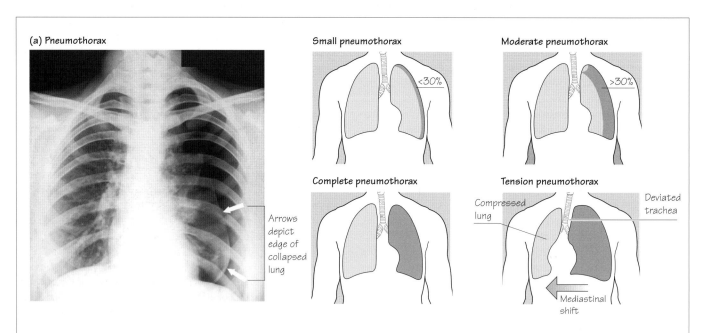

(a) Pneumothorax

Arrows depict edge of collapsed lung

Small pneumothorax
<30%

Moderate pneumothorax
>30%

Complete pneumothorax

Tension pneumothorax
Compressed lung
Deviated trachea
Mediastinal shift

(b)

Management	Degree of collapse		
	Complete	Moderate	Small
Primary	Aspirate/ chest drain	Aspirate	Observe
Secondary	Chest drain	Chest drain	Chest drain
Traumatic/ Iatrogenic	Chest drain	Chest drain	Observe/ chest drain

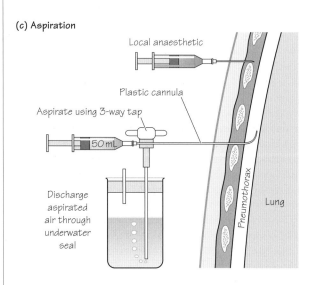

(c) Aspiration

Local anaesthetic

Plastic cannula

Aspirate using 3-way tap

50 mL

Discharge aspirated air through underwater seal

Pneumothorax

Lung

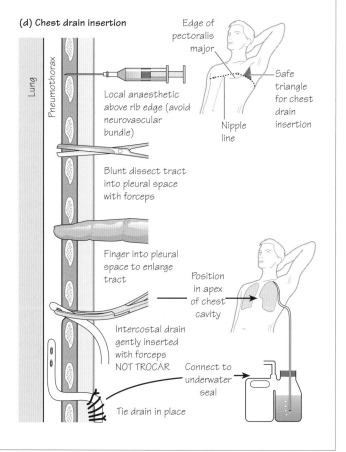

(d) Chest drain insertion

Lung

Pneumothorax

Local anaesthetic above rib edge (avoid neurovascular bundle)

Blunt dissect tract into pleural space with forceps

Finger into pleural space to enlarge tract

Intercostal drain gently inserted with forceps NOT TROCAR

Tie drain in place

Edge of pectoralis major

Safe triangle for chest drain insertion

Nipple line

Position in apex of chest cavity

Connect to underwater seal

A pneumothorax is a collection of air between the visceral and parietal pleura causing a real rather than potential pleural space. Recognition and early drainage can be life saving. Predisposing and precipitating factors include necrotizing lung pathology, chest trauma, ventilator-associated lung injury and cardiothoracic surgery.

Pneumothorax classification

Primary spontaneous pneumothorax (PSP)

This is caused by rupture of small apical subpleural air-cysts ('blebs') but rarely causes significant physiological disturbance. Tall young (20–40 years old) men (M : F 5 : 1) with no underlying lung disease are usually affected. It is the most common type of pneumothorax (prevalence $8/10^5$/year, rising to $200/10^5$/year in subjects >1.9 m in height). Following a second PSP, recurrence is likely (>60%). Pleurodesis to fuse the visceral and parietal pleura using medical (e.g. pleural insertion of bleomycin or talc) or surgical (e.g. abrasion of the pleural lining) means is recommended.

Secondary pneumothorax (SP)

This is associated with respiratory diseases that damage lung architecture, most commonly obstructive (e.g. chronic obstructive pulmonary disease (COPD), asthma), fibrotic or infective (e.g. pneumonia), and occasionally rare or inherited disorders (e.g. Marfan's, cystic fibrosis). The incidence of SP increases with age and the severity of the underlying lung disease. These patients usually require hospital admission as even a small SP in a patient with reduced respiratory reserve may have more serious implications than a large PSP. ICU patients with lung disease are at particular risk of SP due to the high pressures ('barotrauma') and alveolar over-distention ('volutrauma') associated with mechanical ventilation. 'Protective' ventilation strategies using low pressure, limited volume ventilation reduce this risk.

Traumatic (iatrogenic) pneumothorax

This follows blunt (e.g. road traffic accidents) or penetrating (e.g. fractured ribs, stab wounds) chest trauma. Therapeutic procedures (e.g. line insertion, thoracic surgery) are common causes of iatrogenic pneumothorax.

Tension pneumothorax

A **tension pneumothorax** may complicate PSP or SP but is most common during mechanical ventilation and following traumatic pneumothorax. It occurs when air accumulates in the pleural cavity faster than it can be removed. Increased intrathoracic pressure causes mediastinal shift, compression of functioning lung, inhibition of venous return and shock due to reduced cardiac output. It is a medical emergency and fatal if not rapidly relieved by drainage. Detection is a clinical diagnosis; awaiting chest X-ray (CXR) confirmation may be life-threatening. Immediate drainage with a 14 G needle in the second intercostal space in the midclavicular line is essential. A characteristic 'hiss' of escaping gas confirms the diagnosis. A chest drain is then inserted.

Clinical assessment

Pneumothorax is graded and treated according to Fig. 33a and Table b. Sudden breathlessness and/or sharp pleuritic pain suggest a pneumothorax. Most PSPs are small (<30%) and cause few symptoms other than pain. Clinical signs can be surprisingly difficult to detect, but in larger pneumothoraxes reduced air entry and hyper-resonant percussion over one hemithorax are characteristic and may be associated with tachypnoea and cyanosis. Cardiorespiratory compromise may develop remarkably quickly in a tension pneumothorax and requires immediate drainage. Occasionally, other pulmonary air leaks may occur (see below). **Monitoring:** reveals tachycardia, hypotension and desaturation. **Blood gases:** may demonstrate respiratory failure. **CXR:** confirms the diagnosis (Fig. 33a). **Computed tomography (CT) scan:** may detect localized pneumothoraxes.

Management

Immediate supportive therapy includes supplemental oxygen and analgesia. Treatment is dependent on the cause, size and symptoms.

A tension pneumothorax must be drained immediately. A small PSP (<30%) is simply observed and spontaneous reabsorption is confirmed on serial outpatient CXR. A PSP >30% may be aspirated through a 16 G needle in the second intercostal space in the midclavicular line using a 50 mL syringe connected to a three-way tap and underwater seal (Fig. 33c). Following overnight observation, successful aspiration is confirmed by lung re-expansion on repeat CXR. Occasionally, intercostal tube drainage is required for a large PSP with respiratory failure or if aspiration is unsuccessful.

In general, SP and traumatic pneumothoraxes *always* require hospital admission and intercostal chest drain insertion (Fig. 33d). Multiple intercostals drains may be needed to ensure adequate lung re-expansion in some patients with multiple loculated pneumothoraces. In mechanically ventilated patients, high airways pressures or large tidal volumes encourage persistent leaks and must be avoided.

Small chest drains (16 G) are nearly always adequate. Large chest drains are painful and have no significant benefits.

A persistent drain leak suggests development of a **bronchopleural fistula** (BPF). High flow, wall suction with pressures of 5–50 cmH$_2$O, may oppose visceral and parietal pleura allowing spontaneous pleurodesis. Physiotherapy and bronchial toilette is required to maintain airway patency. Early advice on surgical BPF management is essential. Video-assisted thoracoscopy is as effective as thoracotomy at correcting BPF but causes less respiratory dysfunction.

Chest drains are removed when CXR confirms lung expansion and there has been no air leakage through the drain for >24 hours. Drains should not be clamped before removal. Following adequate analgesia, the drain is pulled out when the patient is in inspiration. Purse string sutures around the drainage site are then tightly secured.

Air leaks

Pneumomediastinum describes air in the mediastinal–pleural reflection, outlining the heart and great vessels on CXR. Air may also dissect along perivascular sheaths into the neck causing **subcutaneous emphysema (SE)** or around the heart with **pneumopericardium**, which may cause tamponade. Air leaks follow traumatic damage to the trachea, bronchus and oesophagus or ventilator-induced barotrauma. SE may cause localized cervical or grotesque facial and body swelling. It has a characteristic crackling sensation on palpation. The voice may have a nasal quality and auscultation over the precordium may reveal a 'crunch' with each heart beat (Homan's sign). Management includes good drainage of pneumothorax and 'protective' ventilation strategies (Chapter 41). Failure of spontaneous resolution should prompt investigation, including bronchoscopy, for problems that decrease chest drain efficiency or undetected air leaks.

(a) Pneumonia affecting the right lower lobe

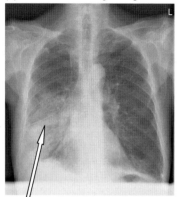

Consolidation right lower lobe

(b) Pneumonia affecting lingula lobe

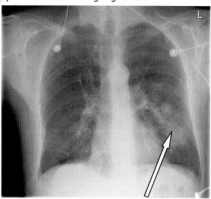

Consolidation lingula lobe

Table 2. Risk factors for pneumonia

Age: >65, <5 years old
Chronic disease (e.g. renal, lung)
Diabetes mellitus
Immunosuppression (e.g. drugs, HIV)
Alcohol dependency
Aspiration (e.g. epilepsy)
Recent viral illness (e.g. influenza)
Malnutrition
Mechanical ventilation
Postoperative (e.g. obesity, smoking)
Environmental (e.g. psittacosis)
Occupational (e.g. Q fever)
Travel abroad (e.g. paragonimiasis)
Air-conditioning (e.g. Legionella)

Table 1. Microorganisms and pathological insults that cause pneumonia

Bacterial infections	Atypical infections	Fungal infection
Streptococcus pneumoniae	Mycoplasma pneumoniae	Aspergillus
Haemophilus influenzae	Legionella pneumophila	Histoplasmosis
Klebsiella pneumoniae	Coxiella burnetii	Candida
Pseudomonas aeruginosa	Chlamydia psittaci	Nocardia
Gram negative (E. coli)		
Viral infections	**Protozoal infections**	**Other causes**
Influenza	Pneumocystis carinii	Aspiration
Coxsackie	Toxoplasmosis	Lipoid pneumonia
Adenovirus	Amoebiasis	Bronchiectasis
Respiratory syncytial	Paragonimiasis	Cystic fibrosis
Cytomegalovirus		Radiation

(c) Non-hospital (i.e. community) management of CAP using the recently validated CRB-65 score

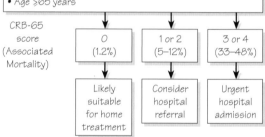

Score 1 point for each of:
• Confusion (mental test score <8 or new disorientation)
• Respiratory rate ≥30/min
• Blood pressure (SBP<90 mmHg or DBP ≤60 mmHg)
• Age ≥65 years

CRB-65 score (Associated Mortality)

0 (1.2%)	1 or 2 (5–12%)	3 or 4 (33–48%)
Likely suitable for home treatment	Consider hospital referral	Urgent hospital admission

(e) Complications and infection specific features of pneumonia

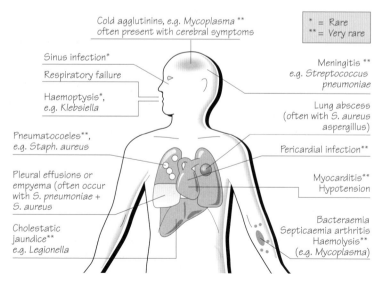

* = Rare
** = Very rare

Cold agglutinins, e.g. Mycoplasma ** often present with cerebral symptoms

Sinus infection*

Respiratory failure

Haemoptysis*, e.g. Klebsiella

Meningitis ** e.g. Streptococcus pneumoniae

Lung abscess (often with S. aureus aspergillus)

Pneumatocoeles**, e.g. Staph. aureus

Pericardial infection**

Pleural effusions or empyema (often occur with S. pneumoniae + S. aureus)

Myocarditis** Hypotension

Cholestatic jaundice** e.g. Legionella

Bacteraemia Septicaemia arthritis Haemolysis** (e.g. Mycoplasma)

(d) Management of CAP in patients admitted to hospital using the recently validated CURB-65 score

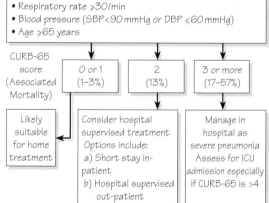

Score 1 point for each of:
• Confusion (mental test score <8 or new disorientation)
• Urea >7mmol/L (i.e. includes use of laboratory tests)
• Respiratory rate ≥30/min
• Blood pressure (SBP<90 mmHg or DBP ≤60 mmHg)
• Age ≥65 years

CURB-65 score (Associated Mortality)

0 or 1 (1–3%)	2 (13%)	3 or more (17–57%)
Likely suitable for home treatment	Consider hospital supervised treatment Options include: a) Short stay in-patient b) Hospital supervised out-patient	Manage in hospital as severe pneumonia Assess for ICU admission especially if CURB-65 is >4

Pneumonia is an **acute lower respiratory tract (LRT) illness**, usually due to **infection**, associated with **fever, focal chest symptoms (± signs)** and **new shadowing on chest X-ray (CXR)** (Fig. 34a). Table 1 lists microorganisms and pathological insults that cause pneumonia.

Classification

In the clinical situation, **microbiological classification** of pneumonia is not practical as causative organisms may not be identified or diagnosis takes several days. Likewise, **anatomical** (radiographical) appearance (e.g. lobar pneumonia (affecting one lobe) or bronchopneumonia (widespread, patchy involvement)) gives little practical information about cause. The following classification is widely accepted.

• **Community acquired pneumonia (CAP):** describes LRT infections occurring within 48 hours of hospital admission in patients who have not been hospitalized for >14 days. The most frequently identified organism is *Streptococcus pneumoniae* (20–75%). *Mycoplasma pneumoniae*, *Chlamydia pneumoniae* and *Legionalla* spp, the 'atypical' bacterial pathogens (2–25%) and viral infections (8–12%) are relatively common causes. *Haemophilus influenzae* and *M. catarrhalis* are associated with COPD exacerbations and staphylococcal infection may follow influenza. Alcoholic, diabetic and nursing-home patients are prone to staphylococcal, anaerobic and Gram-negative organisms.

• **Hospital acquired (nosocomial) pneumonia** (Chapter 35): any LRT infections developing >2 days after hospital admission. Likely organisms are Gram-negative bacilli (~70%) or staphylococcus (~15%).

• **Aspiration/anaerobic pneumonia:** bacteroides and other anaerobic infections follow aspiration of oropharyngeal contents (e.g. CVA).

• **Opportunistic pneumonia** (Chapter 37): immunosuppressed patients (e.g. steroids, chemotherapy, HIV) are susceptible to viral, fungal and mycobacterial infections, in addition to other bacterial organisms.

• **Recurrent pneumonia:** due to aerobic and anaerobic organisms occurs in cystic fibrosis and bronchiectasis.

Epidemiology

Annual incidence: 5–11 cases per 1000 adult population; 15–45% require hospitalization (1–4 cases per 1000) of whom 5–10% are treated in ICU. Incidence is highest in the very young and elderly. **Mortality:** 5–12% in hospitalized patients; 25–50% in ICU patients. **Seasonal variation:** with peaks (e.g. *Mycoplasma* in autumn, *Staphylococcus* in spring) and annual cycles occur (e.g. 4-yearly *Mycoplasma* epidemics). Frequent viral infections increase CAP in winter.

Risk factors

Factors associated with increased risk of CAP are listed in Table 2. **Specific risk factors** include **age** (e.g. *Mycoplasma* in young adults); **occupation** (e.g. brucellosis in abattoir workers, Q fever in sheep workers); **environment** (e.g. psittacosis with pet birds, erlichiosis due to tick bites); or **geographical** (e.g. coccidomycosis in southwest USA). Epidemics of *Coxiella burnetti* (Q fever) or *Legionella pneumophila* are often localized (e.g. Legionnaire's disease may involve a specific hotel due to air-conditioner contamination).

Diagnosis

The aims are to establish the **diagnosis**, identify **complications**, assess **severity** and determine **classification** to aid antibiotic choice.

Clinical features

These are inaccurate without a CXR and cannot predict causative organisms (i.e. 'atypical' pathogens do not have characteristic presentations). **Symptoms** may be general (e.g. malaise, fever, rigors, myalgia) or chest specific (e.g. dyspnoea, pleurisy, cough, haemopty-sis). **Signs** include cyanosis, tachycardia and tachypnoea; with focal dullness, crepitations, bronchial breathing and pleuritic rub on chest examination. In young or old patients and atypical pneumonias (e.g. *Mycoplasma*), **non-respiratory features** (e.g. confusion, rashes, diarrhoea) may predominate. **Complications** are shown in Fig. 34e.

Investigations

Routine blood tests: white cell count (WCC) and C-reactive protein confirm infection; haemolysis and cold agglutinins occur in ~50% of *Mycoplasma* infection; abnormal liver function tests suggest *Legionella* or *Mycoplasma* infection. **Blood gases:** identify respiratory failure. **Microbiology:** no microorganism is isolated in ~33–50% of patients due to previous antibiotic therapy or inadequate specimen collection. Blood cultures in severe CAP, and sputum, pleural fluid and bronchoalveolar lavage samples, with appropriate staining, culture and assessment of antibiotic sensitivity, may determine the pathogen and effective therapy. **Serology:** identifies *Mycoplasma* infection but long processing times limit clinical value. Rapid antigen detection tests for *Legionella* (e.g. urine) and pneumococcus (e.g. serum, pleural fluid) are more useful. **Radiology:** CXR (Fig. 34a) and CT scans aid diagnosis and detect complications.

Severity assessment

The following features are associated with increased mortality and indicate the need for monitoring in ICU: **Clinical:** age >60 years; respiratory rate >30/min; diastolic blood pressure <60 mmHg; new atrial fibrillation; confusion; multilobar involvement; and coexisting illness; **Laboratory:** urea >7 mmol/L; albumin <35 g/L; hypoxaemia P_O_2 < 8 kPa; leucopenia (WCC < 4×10^9/L); leucocytosis (WCC > 20×10^9/L); and bacteraemia. **Severity scoring:** CRB-65 and CURB-65 scores, allocate points for **c**onfusion; **u**rea >7 mmol/L; **r**espiratory rate >30/min; low systolic (<90 mmHg) or diastolic (<60 mmHg) **b**lood pressure and age >**65** years, to stratify patients into mortality groups suitable for different management pathways (Fig. 34c,d).

Management

Supportive measures: include oxygen to maintain $P_aO_2 > 8$ kPa (S_aO_2 < 90%) and intravenous fluid (± inotrope) resuscitation to ensure haemodynamic stability. **Ventilatory support:** non-invasive (e.g. continuous positive airway pressure (CPAP)) or mechanical ventilation may be required in respiratory failure (Chapter 41). **Physiotherapy and bronchoscopy:** aid sputum clearance.

Initial antibiotic therapy: represents the 'best guess', according to pneumonia classification and likely organisms, as microbiological results are not available for 12–72 hours. Therapy is adjusted when results and antibiotic sensitivities become available. The American and British Thoracic Societies (ATS, BTS) recommend the following initial antibiotic protocols for CAP:

• **Non-hospitalized patients:** usually respond to oral therapy with amoxicillin (BTS) or an advanced macrolide (e.g. clarithromycin) or doxycycline (ATS). Patients with severe symptoms or at risk for drug-resistant *S. pneumoniae* (e.g. recent antibiotics, comorbidity) are treated with a beta-lactam plus a macrolide or doxycycline; or an anti-pneumococcal fluoroquinolone (e.g. moxifloxacin) alone.

• **Hospitalized patients:** initial therapy must cover 'atypical' organisms and *S. pneumoniae*. An intravenous macrolide is combined with a beta-lactam or an anti-pneumoccocal fluoroquinolone (ATS/BTS) or cefuroxime (BTS). If not severe, combined ampicillin and macrolide (oral or i.v.) may be adequate (BTS). Staphylococcal infection following influenza and *H. influenzae* in COPD should be covered.

(a) (i) CXR; (ii) CT scan from a patient with hospital acquired pneumonia (HAP) showing consolidation, cavitation and abscess formation

(i)

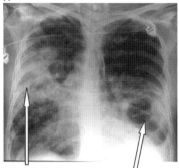

Consolidation

Cavitation

(ii)

Fluid filled abscess

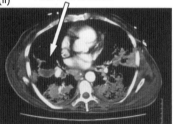

Table 1. Risk factors and modifiable risk factors for HAP and VAP

Un-modifiable risk factors	Modifiable risk factors
1. Host related • Malnutrition • Age: >65, <5 years old • Chronic disease (e.g. renal) • Diabetes • Immunosuppression (e.g. SLE) • Alcohol dependency • Aspiration (e.g. epilepsy) • Recent viral illness • Obesity • Smoking **2. Therapy related** • Mechanical ventilation • Postoperative **3. Epidemiological factors** • Environmental (e.g. psittacosis) • Occupational (e.g. Q fever) • Travel abroad (e.g. paragonomiasis) • Air-conditioning (e.g. Legionella)	**1. Host related** • Nutrition (e.g. enteral feeding) • Pain control, physiotherapy • Limit immunosuppressive therapy • Posture, kinetic beds • Pre-operative smoking cessation **2. Therapy related** • Semi-recumbent position (30° head up) • Early removal of iv lines, ET and NG tubes • minimize sedative use • Avoid gastric overdistention • Avoid intubation + re-intubation • Maintain ET cuff pressure >20 cm H$_2$0* • Subglottic aspiration during intubation • Change + drain ventilator circuits • ? Sucrulfate for stress ulcer prophylaxis **3. Infection control** • Hand washing, sterile technique • Patient isolation • Microbiological surveillance

Table 2. Risk factors for multidrug-resistant pathogens causing hospital acquired pneumonia

• Antimicrobial therapy in the previous 90 days
• Current hospitalization of >5 days
• High frequency of local antibiotic resistance
• Presence of risk factors for HCAP
  Hospitalization for >2 days in the previous 90 days
  Residence in a nursing home
  Home wound care or intravenous therapy
  Chronic dialysis within 30 days
  Family member with MDR pathogen
• Immunosuppressive disease and/or therapy

(b) Pathogenesis of hospital aquired pneumonia

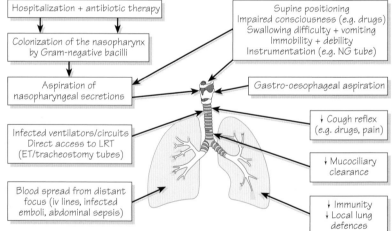

Hospitalization + antibiotic therapy

Colonization of the nasopharynx by Gram-negative bacilli

Aspiration of nasopharyngeal secretions

Infected ventilators/circuits Direct access to LRT (ET/tracheostomy tubes)

Blood spread from distant focus (iv lines, infected emboli, abdominal sepsis)

Supine positioning
Impaired consciousness (e.g. drugs)
Swallowing difficulty + vomiting
Immobility + debility
Instrumentation (e.g. NG tube)

Gastro-oesophageal aspiration

↓ Cough reflex (e.g. drugs, pain)

↓ Mucociliary clearance

↓ Immunity ↓ Local lung defences

(c) Likely pathogens and empirical antibiotic treatment of hospital acquired pneumonias

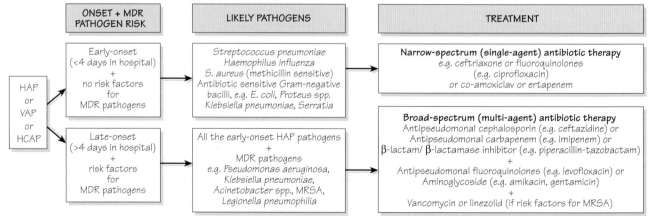

ONSET + MDR PATHOGEN RISK	LIKELY PATHOGENS	TREATMENT
HAP or VAP or HCAP	Early-onset (<4 days in hospital) + no risk factors for MDR pathogens	Streptococcus pneumoniae Haemophilus influenza S. aureus (methicillin sensitive) Antibiotic sensitive Gram-negative bacilli, e.g. E. coli, Proteus spp. Klebsiella pneumoniae, Serratia	**Narrow-spectrum (single-agent) antibiotic therapy** e.g. ceftriaxone or fluoroquinolones (e.g. ciprofloxacin) or co-amoxiclav or ertapenem
	Late-onset (>4 days in hospital) + risk factors for MDR pathogens	All the early-onset HAP pathogens + MDR pathogens e.g. Pseudomonas aeruginosa, Klebsiella pneumoniae, Acinetobacter spp., MRSA, Legionella pneumophilia	**Broad-spectrum (multi-agent) antibiotic therapy** Antipseudomonal cephalosporin (e.g. ceftazidine) or Antipseudomonal carbapenem (e.g. imipenem) or β-lactam/ β-lactamase inhibitor (e.g. piperacillin-tazobactam) + Antipseudomonal fluoroquinolones (e.g. levofloxacin) or Aminoglycoside (e.g. amikacin, gentamicin) + Vancomycin or linezolid (if risk factors for MRSA)

Hospital acquired (nosocomial) pneumonia (HAP) including **ventilator associated pneumonia (VAP)** and **healthcare-associated pneumonia (HCAP)** affects 0.5–2% of hospital patients and is a leading cause of nosocomial infection (i.e. with wound, urinary tract, blood stream). Pathogenesis, causative organisms and outcome differ from community acquired pneumonia (CAP). Preventative measures and early antibiotic therapy, guided by awareness of the role of multidrug resistant (MDR) pathogens, improves outcome.

Definitions

HAP: pulmonary infection developing >48 hours after hospital admission that was not incubating at the time of admission. **VAP:** pneumonia developing >48–72 hours after endotracheal intubation. **HCAP:** includes any patient admitted to hospital for >2 days within 90 days of the infection, residing in a nursing home, receiving therapy (e.g. wound care, intravenous therapy) within 30 days of the current infection, or attending a hospital or haemodialysis clinic.

Epidemiology

Incidence: varies between 5 and 10 episodes per 1000 discharges and is highest on surgical and ICU wards and in teaching hospitals. It lengthens hospital stay by between 3 and 14 days per patient. The risk of HAP increases 6–20-fold during mechanical ventilation (MV) and in ICU, it accounts for 25% of infections and ~50% of prescribed antibiotics. VAP accounts for >80% of all HAP and occurs in 9–27% of intubated patients. **Risk factors:** include those that predispose to CAP and factors associated with HAP pathogenesis, some of which can be **prevented** (Table 1). **Mortality:** between 30% and 70%. **Early onset HAP/VAP** (<4 days in hospital) is usually caused by antibiotic-sensitive bacteria and carries a better prognosis than **late onset HAP/VAP** (>4 days in hospital), which is associated with MDR pathogens. In early onset HAP/VAP, prior antibiotic therapy or hospitalization predisposes to MDR pathogens and is treated as late onset HAP/VAP. Bacteraemia, medical rather than surgical illness, VAP and late or ineffective antibiotic therapy also increase mortality.

Pathogenesis (Fig. 35b)

Oropharyneal colonization with enteric Gram-negative bacteria occurs in most hospital patients due to immobility, impaired consciousness, instrumentation (e.g. nasogastric tubes), poor hygiene or inhibition of gastric acid secretion. Subsequent aspiration of nasopharyngeal secretions (± gastric contents) causes HAP (Fig. 35b).

Aetiology

Time of onset (early/late) and risk factors for infection with MDR organisms (Table 2) determine potential pathogens (Fig. 35c). Aerobic Gram-negative bacilli (e.g. *Klebsiella pneumoniae, Pseudomonas aeruginosa, Escherichia coli*) cause ~60–70% of infections and *Staphylococcus aureus* ~10–15%. *S. pneumoniae* and *H. influenza* may be isolated in early onset HAP/VAP. In ICU, >50% *S. aureus* infections are methicillin resistant (MRSA). *S. aureus* is more common in diabetics and ICU patients.

Diagnosis

Requires both *clinical* and *microbiological* assessment. It may be difficult as: (i) clinical features are non-specific or confused with concurrent illness (e.g. acute respiratory distress syndrome (ARDS)); and (ii) previous antibiotics limit microbiological evaluation. **Clinical:** HAP is suspected when new radiographical infiltrates occur with features suggestive of infection (e.g. fever >38°C, purulent sputum, leucocytosis, hypoxaemia). **Diagnostic tests:** confirm infection and determine the causative organism (± antibiotic sensitivity). They include routine blood counts, blood gases, serology, blood cultures, pleural effusions aspiration, sputum, endotracheal aspirate and bronchioalveolar lavage microbiology and CXR. CT scanning (Fig. 35a) aids diagnosis and detects **complications** (e.g. abscesses).

Management

Early diagnosis and treatment improves morbidity and mortality and requires constant vigilance in hospital patients. Antibiotic therapy must not be delayed while awaiting microbiological results.

Supportive therapy

This includes supplemental **oxygen** to maintain $P_aO_2 > 8\,kPa$ ($S_aO_2 < 90\%$), **intravenous fluids (± vasopressors/inotropes)** for haemodynamic stability and **ventilatory support** (e.g. continuous positive airway pressure (CPAP), MV) in respiratory failure. **Physiotherapy** and **analgesia** aid sputum clearance postoperatively and in the immobilized patient. **Semi-recumbent** (i.e. 30° bed-head elevation) nursing of bed-bound patients reduces aspiration risk. Strict glycaemic control and attention to other modifiable risk factors (Table 1) may improve outcome.

Antibiotic therapy

This is empirical while awaiting microbiological guidance. The key decision is whether the patient has risk factors for MDR organisms. Figure 35c illustrates the ATS guidelines for initial, i.v antibiotic therapy. Local patterns of antibiotic resistance are used to modify these protocols.

• In **early onset HAP/VAP** with no risk factors for MDR organisms, **monotherapy** with a beta-lactam/beta-lactamase, third-generation cephalosporin or fluoroquinolone antibiotic is advised.

• In **late onset HAP/VAP** with risk factors for MDR pathogens (Table 2), **combination therapy**, with broad-spectrum antibiotics to cover MDR Gram-negative bacilli and MRSA (e.g. vancomycin) is required (Fig. 35c). Adjunctive therapy with inhaled aminoglycosides or polymyxin is considered in patients not improving with systemic therapy.

A short course of therapy (e.g. 7 days) is appropriate if the clinical response is good. Aggressive or resistant pathogens (e.g. *P. aeruginosa, S. aureus*) may require 14–21 days' treatment. Therapy is focused on causative organisms when culture data are available and unnecessary antibiotics withdrawn. Sterile cultures (in the absence of new antibiotics for >72 hours) virtually rules out HAP.

Other pneumonias

Aspiration/anaerobic pneumonia: *Bacteroides* and other anaerobic infections follow aspiration of oropharyngeal contents due to laryngeal incompetence or reduced consciousness (e.g. cerebrovascular accident; CVA, drugs). Lung abscesses are common. Antibiotic therapy should include anaerobic coverage (e.g. metronidazole).

Pneumonia during immunosuppression (Chapter 37): HIV, transplant and chemotherapy patients are susceptible to viral (e.g. cytomegalovirus), fungal (e.g. *Aspergillus*) and mycobacterial infections, in addition to the normal range of organisms. HIV patients with CD4 counts <200/mm^3, also develop opportunistic infections such as *Pneumocystis carinii* pneumonia (PCP) or toxoplasma. Severely immunocompromised patients require broad-spectrum antibiotic, antifungal and antiviral regimens. PCP is treated with steroids and high dose co-trimoxazole.

(a)

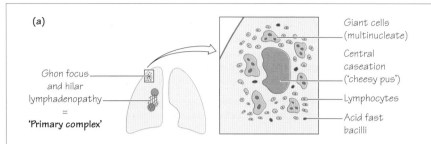

Ghon focus and hilar lymphadenopathy = 'Primary complex'

Giant cells (multinucleate)

Central caseation ('cheesy pus')

Lymphocytes

Acid fast bacilli

(b) CXR of patients with TB

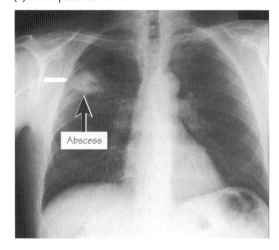

Abscess

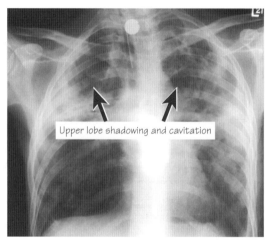

Upper lobe shadowing and cavitation

Tuberculosis

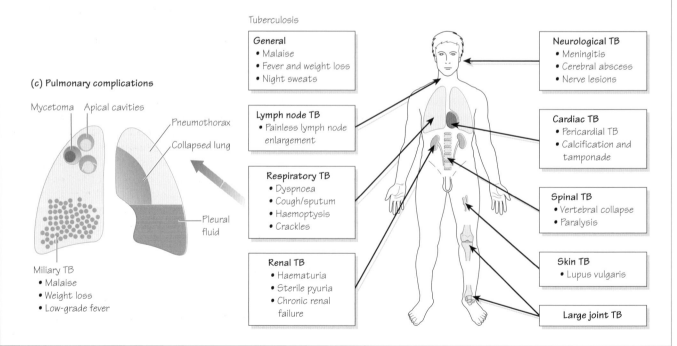

(c) Pulmonary complications

Mycetoma   Apical cavities

Pneumothorax

Collapsed lung

Pleural fluid

Miliary TB
• Malaise
• Weight loss
• Low-grade fever

General
• Malaise
• Fever and weight loss
• Night sweats

Lymph node TB
• Painless lymph node enlargement

Respiratory TB
• Dyspnoea
• Cough/sputum
• Haemoptysis
• Crackles

Renal TB
• Haematuria
• Sterile pyuria
• Chronic renal failure

Neurological TB
• Meningitis
• Cerebral abscess
• Nerve lesions

Cardiac TB
• Pericardial TB
• Calcification and tamponade

Spinal TB
• Vertebral collapse
• Paralysis

Skin TB
• Lupus vulgaris

Large joint TB

Worldwide, tuberculosis (TB) affects 10 million people and causes 3 million deaths each year. In developed countries it is uncommon, affecting ~1 per 10 000 population. Pulmonary TB is most common in Asian, Chinese and West Indian people. Airborne transmission and close contact spread the disease. Those who are elderly, malnourished or immunosuppressed (HIV infection, diabetes mellitus, corticosteroid therapy, alcoholism, intercurrent lymphoma) are more susceptible. Improved housing and nutrition reduce incidence.

Pathogenesis

Primary pulmonary TB is caused by the acid-fast bacillus *Mycobacterium tuberculosis*. The inhaled bacillus infects well-ventilated, poorly perfused upper lung lobes subpleurally. A **granuloma** forms (Fig. 36a) known as the **Ghon focus**, and with the enlarged hilar lymph nodes draining the affected lung is known as the 'primary complex' (Fig. 36a). This occurs over 3–8 weeks, and is accompanied by development of an inflammatory reaction to injection of tubercular protein (**tuberculin**) into the skin, which can be used as a diagnostic test (**Mantoux** or **Heaf** test). Complete healing usually follows, with fibrosis and calcification of the Ghon focus and immunity to further infection.

Post-primary pulmonary TB occurs if the Ghon focus fails to heal due to poor host defences, or following reactivation. It is potentially fatal. Local dissemination causes **tuberculous pneumonia** and **pleural effusions**. Bloodborne spread may affect the meninges or individual organs. In a few cases, widespread infection involves many tissues (**miliary TB**).

Clinical features

Primary pulmonary TB usually occurs at an early age. Often asymptomatic with no clinical signs, it may cause a mild febrile illness, **erythema nodosum** (painful, indurated shin lesions) and small pleural effusions. Bronchial compression by lymphadenopathy may cause wheeze and occasionally lobar collapse followed by late **bronchiectasis** (Chapter 32).

Post-primary TB develops over months, with malaise, anorexia, weight loss, night sweats and a productive cough. Breathlessness, chest pain, haemoptysis and cervical lymphadenopathy may occur. Clinical signs of pneumonia and pleural effusion are common, whereas lupus vulgaris (an indolent skin infection) is less frequent. **Miliary TB** presents with a non-specific pyrexial illness, malaise and weight loss. Sparse clinical signs include hepatomegaly and choroidal tubercles in the retina.

Investigation

Blood tests may detect anaemia, decreased sodium and increased calcium.

Mantoux test: strongly positive in post-primary pulmonary TB (>5 mm skin induration with 10 units of intradermal tuberculin; read at 3 days). Often negative in miliary TB (reduced host response) and HIV (reduced cellular immunity).

Heaf test (screening test; now less commonly used): a ring of six pinpricks is made through a tuberculin solution on the forearm. No response at 4–7 days (grade 0) demonstrates lack of immunity; 4–6 discrete nodules (grade 1) or a ring formed by coalition of all pinpricks (grade 2) indicate immunity. A single nodule formed by infilling of the ring (grade 3) represents recent contact or early tuberculous infection, and a nodule >5–7 mm with surface vesicles or ulceration (grade 4) suggests infection.

Microbiology: the acid-fast bacilli may be detected in sputum or lung washings using Ziehl–Neelsen stain. However, bacilli are slow-growing, and culture and drug sensitivities take 4–6 weeks. Bone marrow or cerebrospinal fluid (CSF) culture may confirm the diagnosis of miliary TB.

Histopathology: pleural aspiration with biopsy confirms TB in ~90% of patients with pleural effusions. Liver biopsy will isolate miliary TB in ~60% of cases.

Chest radiography (Fig. 36b): upper lobe shadowing is suggestive. Apical cavities, pleural effusions and pneumothoraces may occur. In miliary TB, widespread small nodules (2–3 mm diameter) are diffusely spread throughout the lungs (miliary shadowing), and are easily missed.

Drug therapy

Prognosis is good if the patient is not immunocompromised. Good nutrition, reduced alcohol consumption and **compliance with drug therapy** are important factors. Uncomplicated pulmonary TB is treated for 6 months. Initially, at least three drugs are used, to prevent development of resistant strains. The recommended regimen is rifampicin, pyrazinamide and isoniazid for 2 months, followed by rifampicin and isoniazid for 4 months. Additional pyridoxine prevents isoniazid-induced peripheral neuropathy. Liver function should be monitored, as rifampicin and pyrazinamide can cause liver dysfunction. If drug resistance is suspected (TB recurrence in a non-compliant patient) then a four-drug regimen (adding ethambutol) may be initiated. When culture results are available, alternative drugs replace those to which the mycobacterium is not sensitive. Ethambutol (monitor colour vision for optic neuritis), streptomycin (monitor plasma levels to avoid hearing impairment) or ciprofloxacin may be used. In severe pulmonary TB, corticosteroids occasionally improve results.

In some organs (e.g. bone), TB is treated for longer, often with additional drugs. In meningeal or cerebral TB, a four-drug regimen for 12 months with additional steroids is recommended, to ensure adequate brain penetration and to prevent cranial nerve compression by meningeal scarring.

Complications

Reactivation of old tuberculous scars may occur when a patient is immunocompromised (Fig. 36c). Chemoprophylaxis with isoniazid is often given before immunosuppressive treatment (chemotherapy, organ transplantation). Bronchiectasis and lung cavities with secondary fungal infections (mycetoma), cranial nerve lesions and renal tract obstructions may develop due to scarring associated with healing after TB. Non-compliance or inadequate treatment results in multiresistant strains of mycobacteria that may be very difficult to eradicate. Compulsory supervision and isolation of these patients may be required.

Prevention and contact tracing

Vaccination of non-immune subjects with **BCG** (bacille Calmette–Guérin), a non-virulent strain of bovine TB, produces immunity and reduces the risk of pulmonary TB by 70%. Community health services **must be notified** when a patient is diagnosed with TB, to trace contacts and prevent spread. Contacts are screened with a Heaf test. If this suggests a risk of infection, then chest radiography and appropriate follow-up is arranged.

Respiratory infections in HIV infection

(a) Common respiratory infections in HIV-infected individuals

Microbe	Typical CD4$^+$ cell count (per mm^3)
Bacteria	
S. pneumoniae	Any
Haemophilus species	Any
P. aeruginosa	<200
L. pneumophila	Any
Mycobacteria	
M. tuberculosis	Any (extrapulmonary or atypical presentation when <200)
Disseminated MAC	<50
Fungi	
Pneumocystis carinii	<200
Cryptococcus neoformans	<200
Histoplasma capsulatum	<200
Coccidiodes immitis	<100
Virus	
Cytomegalovirus	<50

(b) CXR of *Pneumocystis carinii* pneumonia, showing diffuse alveolar infiltrate

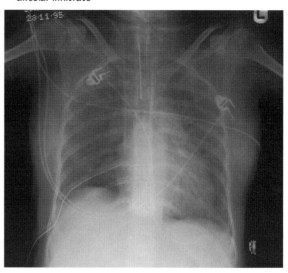

Acquired immune deficiency syndrome (AIDS) is caused by human immunodeficiency virus (**HIV**) which impairs and depletes CD4+ T lymphocytes (Chapter 18). Failure of T lymphocyte function predisposes to viral or fungal infections, and neoplasia. Highly active antiretroviral therapy (**HAART**) allows expansion of the immune system and improves survival of patients with AIDS, partly by decreasing the rate of respiratory infection. Nevertheless, HIV-infected individuals are at increased risk of infection with common bacteria, **mycobacteria (TB),** *Pneumocystis carinii* or **other fungi** (Fig. 37a).

Pneumocystis carinii **pneumonia (PCP)** is most common, although incidence has decreased with **co-trimoxazole prophylaxis**. PCP seems to be a disease of developed countries—it rarely occurs in Africa. **Clinical features** include progressive dyspnoea on exertion, malaise, fever, non-productive cough and hypoxia. In the HIV-infected patient, PCP is indolent over weeks. **Pneumothorax** (Chapter 33) occurs in 2% of cases, particularly in patients receiving aerosolized prophylaxis. Chest X-ray (CXR) usually shows diffuse interstitial infiltrates (Fig. 37b). Demonstration of **pneumocysts** or **trophozoites** in induced sputum or bronchoalveolar lavage is diagnostic in ~90% of cases. High-dose intravenous **co-trimoxazole** is the most effective therapy. Corticosteroids reduce alveolitis, respiratory failure and mortality.

Bacterial pneumonias (Chapters 34 & 35) are extremely common in HIV-infected patients. The presence of high fever, purulent sputum, rapid onset of symptoms or pleuritic chest pain help distinguish bacterial pneumonia from PCP. *Legionella* infections are more common in patients with HIV infection.

Tuberculosis (Chapter 36) is a significant concern; ~33% of HIV-infected patients exposed to *Mycobacterium tuberculosis* develop primary disease, and patients with prior exposure have a 10% per year chance of reactivation. **Tuberculin tests** should be performed on all HIV patients; evidence of prior infection requires prophylactic treatment in the absence of active disease. Clinical features of TB depend on degree of immunosuppression—as this advances, **mediastinal adenopathy, diffuse or miliary pulmonary infiltrates,** and extrapulmonary involvement become more typical. Patients treated with HAART may develop worsening systemic symptoms due to immune reconstitution. The high prevalence of TB in patients with HIV infection has contributed to the spread of **multidrug resistance**.

HIV-induced immunodeficiency increases risk of infection by **fungi,** many of which are ubiquitous in the environment. *Cryptococcus* often has concurrent respiratory manifestations with meningitis. In endemic areas, **histoplasmosis** and **coccidioidomycosis** may cause respiratory disease in HIV-infected individuals. Diagnosis requires stain or culture of the fungus.

Malignancies involving the respiratory system may be confused with infections in HIV-infected individuals. **Kaposi's sarcoma** (KS) and **non-Hodgkin's lymphoma** (NHL) are the most common. KS is a tumour of vascular origin related to infection with **human herpesvirus 8**. Clinical manifestations range from asymptomatic incidental discovery to fulminant disease causing respiratory failure. NHL typically occurs in patients with advanced immunosuppression and are typically aggressive B cell or Burkitt's lymphoma, suggesting pre-existing herpesvirus infections. HIV infection increases the risk of developing **advanced lung cancer** at young age, with a poor prognosis.

38 Smoking

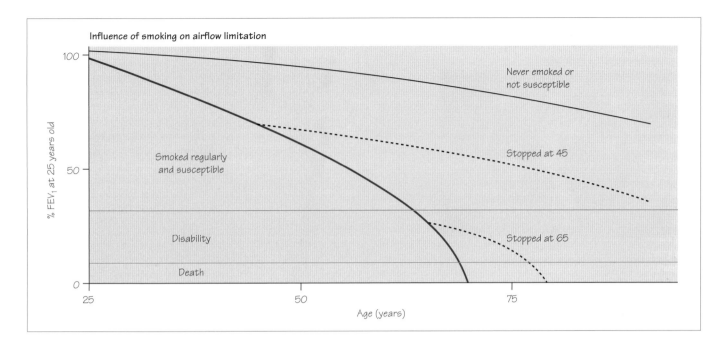

Tobacco use goes back 2000 years, with its initial cultivation in the Americas. During the twentieth century tobacco use became a world-wide public health problem with almost **20 billion cigarettes** being consumed by almost 2 billion individuals. In addition, oral and other smoked forms of tobacco are popular in many parts of the world. It is estimated that tobacco contributes to approximately **5 million deaths per year worldwide** due to its effect on lung cancer, coronary artery diseases and COPD.

Effects: tobacco smoke is comprised of a multitude of gaseous and particulate chemicals with potential effects on the respiratory system. **Carbon monoxide** from incomplete combustion leads to measurable elevations of carboxyhaemoglobin in smokers. **Polycyclic aromatic hydrocarbons** in cigarette smoke have been shown to cause gene mutations that are frequently present in primary lung cancers. Smoke inhalation also has deleterious effects on respiratory **epithelial ciliary function** and **mucociliary transport** (Chapter 18). Cigarette smokers have a greater frequency of acute and chronic morbidity, absenteeism and respiratory symptoms (cough, phlegm, wheeze, dyspnoea) than non-smokers.

Cancer (Chapter 39)
Smoking causes an up to **40-fold increase** in the risk of developing **bronchogenic lung carcinoma** compared to non-smokers who have a less than 1% lifetime risk. The risk is related to exposure as measured in pack-years. Smoking cessation will decrease this risk with time; however, even a decade after quitting, former smokers have approximately twice the risk of lung cancer than those who never smoked.

COPD (Chapter 25)
Cigarette smoking greater than 15 pack-years is the major risk factor for developing **COPD** as defined by a reduction in forced expiratory flow ($FEV_1/FVC <70\%$). Continued smoking causes acceleration in the normal age-related loss of lung function and development of airway hyperreactivity (Fig. 38). Smoking will also worsen symptoms, make treatment more difficult and accelerate loss of lung function in patients with asthma.

Other smoking-related diseases
Community acquired pneumonia is strongly associated with smoking, while smoking is a risk factor for **respiratory bronchiolitis**, **interstitial lung disease** and **eosinophilic granuloma**. Smoking is also a cause of vascular and systemic diseases, particularly **atherosclerotic disease**. Smoking is associated with coronary artery disease, cerebrovascular disease, aortic aneurysm and peripheral vascular disease. Additionally, smoking is associated with **venous thrombotic disease** and **pulmonary embolus** (Chapter 27), particularly in combination with other risks (obesity, contraceptives). Some studies suggest an association between smoking and the development of diabetes, peptic ulcer disease, gastro-oesophageal reflux disease and Crohn's disease. Smoking has also an inverse risk of development and severity of ulcerative colitis.

Maternal smoking during pregnancy or postpartum increases the risk of developing COPD and asthma in the child, independent of personal smoking. **Passive smoking** also is associated with the same risks of disease as first-hand smoking.

Smoking cessation slows disease progression and reverses the risk (Fig. 38). Unfortunately, prolonged quit rates are usually <33%. The most effective programme combines physician advice, nicotine replacement and antidepressant treatment, although informing smokers of abnormalities in diagnostic testing (e.g. spirometry) increases the chance of quitting.

(a) Mass on CT: A >3 cm spiculated mass is seen in upper lobe of the right lung

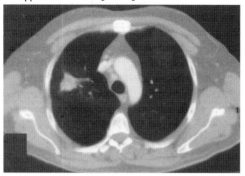

(b) Fibreoptic bronchoscopy showing tumour invading bronchus

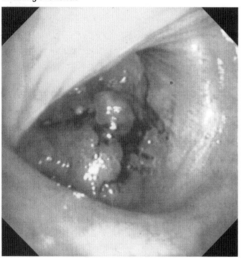

(c) CXR showing squamous cell tumour in hilar region

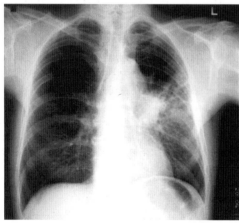

(d) Staging system for non-small cell lung cancers

Stage	T (tumour)	N (node)	M (metastasis)	Key
IA	T1	N0	M0	**T1:** ≤3 cm without division
IB	T2	N0	M0	**T2:** >3 cm, or invasion of main bronchus
IIA	T1	N1	M0	>2 cm from main carina, or invades
IIB	T2	N1	M0	visceral pleura, or bronchus causing
	T3	N0	M0	obstruction
				T3: Invades chest wall or pleura, or main
				bronchus <2 cm from main carina
				T4: Invades adjacent structure,
				malignant effusion, satellite nodules
IIIA	T1, 2, 3	N2	M0	**N0:** No lymph node metastasis
	T3	N1	M0	**N1:** Ipsilateral hilar lymph nodes
IIIB	T1, 2, 3, 4	N3	M0	**N2:** Ipsilateral mediastinal or subcarinal
	T4	N1, 2	M0	lymph nodes
				N3: Contralateral, scalene or supra-
				clavicular lymph nodes
IV	T1–4	N0–3	M1	**M0:** No distant metastasis
				M1: Any distant metastasis

(e) Survival for non-small cell cancer

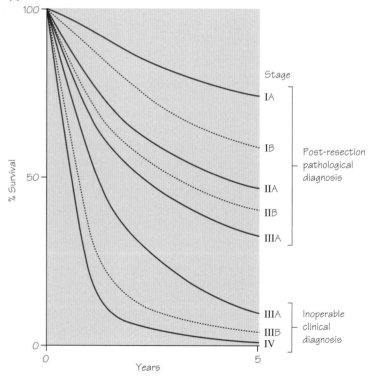

More people die in the USA and Europe from **lung cancer** than from breast, prostate and colon cancer combined. Furthermore, the number of cases is likely to increase in the next 25 years due to continued use of cigarettes, particularly in women. Lung cancer has a **worse prognosis** than other common cancers, with an overall **5-year survival** of **13%**.

Risks

Cigarette smoking accounts for the vast majority of lung cancer cases. Risk is directly related to the duration and number of cigarettes smoked, age of initiation, depth of inhalation and levels of tar and nicotine. In heavy smokers (>20 pack-years) the lifetime risk of lung cancer is 10%, 10–30 times greater than for lifelong non-smokers (<0.3%). After quitting cigarettes, risk gradually declines over 15 years, but remains 2–5 times greater than in non-smokers. **Passive smoking** in non-smokers may increase the risk by ~1.5%.

Asbestos exposure is the most common occupational risk for lung cancer (Chapter 31). Tobacco smoke is synergistic with asbestosis, increasing the relative risk to 6–60 times that of a non-smoker. **Radon gas**, found naturally in rocks, soil and ground water, may also increase risk.

Classification

Lung cancers are divided pathologically into **small cell** (**SC**, 20–30% of total) and **non-small cell** (**NSC**, 70–80% of total) types. **NSC** types are grouped due to their similar biology, treatment and prognosis, and include **squamous cell** (30%), **large cell** (15%) and **adenocarcinoma** (33%), which is increasing in prevalence, especially in women. **Adenocarcinomas** typically present as a peripheral nodule (<3 cm) or mass (>3 cm); they are the most common type in non-smokers, and mainly arise in areas of pulmonary scarring. Bronchoalveolar cell carcinoma is an adenocarcinoma variant with low metastatic potential. **Squamous cell carcinomas** arise from the bronchial epithelium, and generally present as a central mass with tumour visible in the airway (Fig. 39a,b), often with symptoms due to local tumour invasion (cough, haemoptysis, chest pain and hoarseness). **Large cell carcinoma** is undifferentiated, and lacks the histological features of adenocarcinoma or squamous cell carcinoma; it generally presents as a large peripheral mass, often with metastases. **SC** carcinomas arise from neuroendocrine cells in the bronchial submucosa, and typically present as a central mass with lymph node enlargement. These are aggressive tumours that invade lymphatics and blood vessels. Nearly all have metastasized at diagnosis.

Presentation

Less than 10% of lung cancers are discovered incidentally in asymptomatic patients. Most patients are 50–70 years of age, with nonspecific symptoms including new unresolving cough, haemoptysis, chest pain, hoarseness, dyspnoea on exertion, malaise and weight loss. Symptoms due to haematogenous **extrathoracic metastasis** to bone, liver, bone marrow, adrenals and brain are present in around one-third of patients at diagnosis.

Paraneoplastic syndromes—signs or symptoms associated with lung cancers that are not related directly to metastatic tumour—may precede radiographical demonstration. They may be due to secretion of hormones or hormone-like substances from tumours, or serum autoantibodies (e.g. anti-Hu) related to tumour antigens. SC carcinoma is associated with most paraneoplastic syndromes including Cushing's syndrome, syndrome of inappropriate secretion of antidiuretic hormone (SIADH), Lambert–Eaton syndrome, cerebellar ataxia or idiopathic orthostatic hypotension. Squamous cell cancer may cause hypercalcaemia from release of parathyroid hormone-related peptide.

Physical findings in the lung are related to disease extent. Small **parenchymal nodules** are undetectable by physical examination. Focal findings may be due to atelectasis, airway invasion, pleural effusion (Chapter 30) or supraclavicular adenopathy. Invasion of adjacent structures may cause superior vena cava syndrome (obstruction), Horner's syndrome (autonomic overactivity) or brachial plexopathy. Digital clubbing or hypertrophic pulmonary osteoarthropathy may be present.

Evaluation

Evaluation of patients with suspected lung cancer should include demonstration of **malignancy, staging** and **suitability for therapy**. Radiographs provide information regarding the size and location of the tumour, benign calcification, involvement of adjacent structures, atelectasis, pleural effusion and adenopathy (Fig. 39c). **Computed tomography (CT) scans** are superior to plain X-rays. If a focal lesion does not change in 2 years, it is unlikely to be malignant. **Positron emission tomography (PET) scanning** has a high sensitivity for distinguishing benign from malignant nodules and for detecting nodal or distant metastases.

Staging is assessment of the extent of the tumour, and largely determines treatment options and prognosis. Separate staging systems are used for SC and NSC cancers. **SC cancer** is staged as either **limited** or **extensive** disease. **Limited disease** describes tumour confined to one hemithorax, including malignant pleural effusion and supraclavicular lymph node metastasis. **Extensive disease** describes metastatic spread beyond the hemithorax. SC cancer is generally an incurable disease. Standard therapy for limited disease (33%) is combination chemotherapy and radiotherapy, with response rates approaching 90%; median survival with therapy is ~18 months. Standard therapy for extensive disease (66%) is chemotherapy. The response rate is ~70%, treatment prolonging median survival from ~3 months to ~1 year.

NSC cancer staging is based on the **tumour** (T), **node** (N) and **metastasis** (M) classification system (Fig. 39d). **T3** tumours invade thoracic structures that are potentially resectable, and **T4** tumours include malignant effusions or tumours invading non-resectable structures. Summation of **TNM categories** determines the stage of disease and treatment, and predicts survival (Fig. 39e). In functional patients with **stage I** or **II** disease and adequate pulmonary reserve (postoperative FEV_1 >800 mL), **surgical resection** is optimal. Some patients with **stage IIIA** disease are surgical candidates. Patients with **stage IIIB** or **IV** disease are not candidates for curative resection. Unresectable disease is generally treated with **chemotherapy** and **radiation therapy**, or radiation alone. **Stage IV** disease is incurable (median survival 6–12 months). Treatment options are palliative. Painful bone metastases, brain metastasis or airway obstruction may improve with directed therapy. The benefit of aggressive chemotherapy for patients with advanced disease is modest. **Platinum** and **taxol-based** chemotherapy regimens are currently most common for NSC cancer.

Acute respiratory distress syndrome

(a) Acute respiratory distress syndrome

Pathophysiology

Systemic inflammatory response (sepsis/trauma)

Direct alveolar damage (aspiration/pneumonia)

Endotoxin IL-1, IL-6, TNFα → White cell activation

White cell adhesion and migration

IL-1, IL-8 Increased permeability and consolidation

Decreased surfactant with alveolar collapse

H_2O

Alveolar flooding

Endothelial and alveolar cell damage

Loss of surfactant and increased permeability

Widespread alveolar and dependent consolidation

CXR of trauma-induced ARDS

04-05-95

CT scan of ARDS

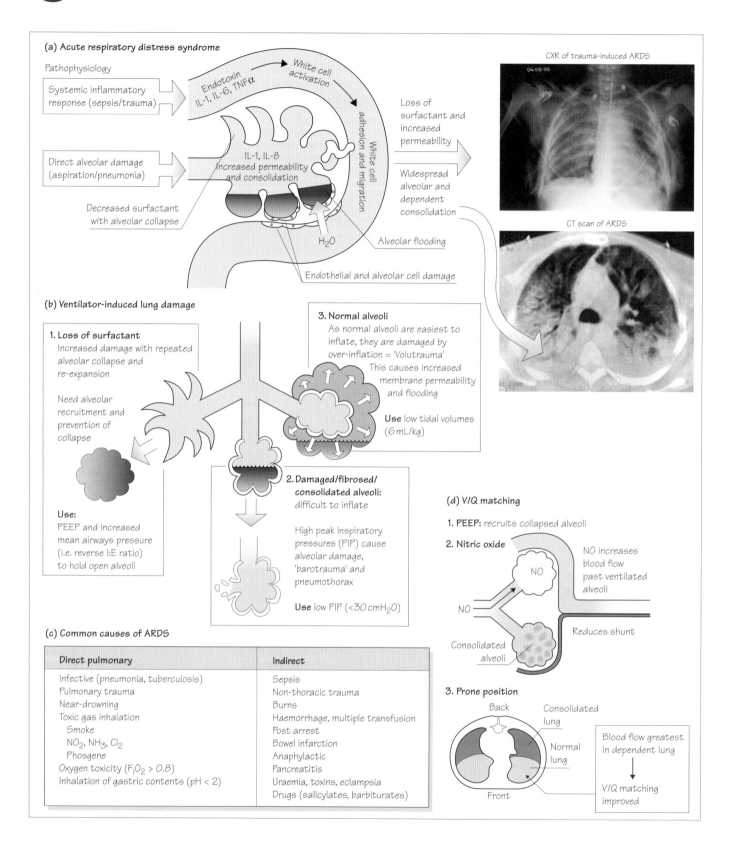

(b) Ventilator-induced lung damage

1. Loss of surfactant
Increased damage with repeated alveolar collapse and re-expansion

Need alveolar recruitment and prevention of collapse

Use:
PEEP and increased mean airways pressure (i.e. reverse I:E ratio) to hold open alveoli

3. Normal alveoli
As normal alveoli are easiest to inflate, they are damaged by over-inflation = 'Volutrauma' This causes increased membrane permeability and flooding

Use low tidal volumes (6 mL/kg)

2. Damaged/fibrosed/ consolidated alveoli: difficult to inflate

High peak inspiratory pressures (PIP) cause alveolar damage, 'barotrauma' and pneumothorax

Use low PIP (<30 cmH$_2$O)

(d) V/Q matching

1. PEEP: recruits collapsed alveoli

2. Nitric oxide

NO

NO

NO increases blood flow past ventilated alveoli

Consolidated alveoli

Reduces shunt

3. Prone position

Back

Consolidated lung

Normal lung

Front

Blood flow greatest in dependent lung
↓
V/Q matching improved

(c) Common causes of ARDS

Direct pulmonary	Indirect
Infective (pneumonia, tuberculosis)	Sepsis
Pulmonary trauma	Non-thoracic trauma
Near-drowning	Burns
Toxic gas inhalation	Haemorrhage, multiple transfusion
Smoke	Post arrest
NO$_2$, NH$_3$, Cl$_2$	Bowel infarction
Phosgene	Anaphylactic
Oxygen toxicity (F$_i$O$_2$ > 0.8)	Pancreatitis
Inhalation of gastric contents (pH < 2)	Uraemia, toxins, eclampsia
	Drugs (salicylates, barbiturates)

Acute respiratory distress syndrome (ARDS) is most simply defined as 'leaky lung syndrome' or 'low pressure (i.e. non-cardiogenic) pulmonary oedema'. It describes an acute, diffuse inflammatory lung injury, often in previously healthy lungs (Fig. 40a) in response to a variety of direct (i.e. inhaled) or indirect (i.e. bloodborne) insults.

The **internationally agreed criteria** for diagnosis of ARDS are:

1 Severe hypoxaemia, P_aO_2/F_iO_2 <200, ($\pm$ positive end-expiratory pressure (PEEP)), e.g. P_aO_2 (55 mmHg)/F_iO_2 (80% inspired O_2) = 55/0.8 = (75)

2 Bilateral diffuse pulmonary infiltrates on chest X-ray

3 Normal or only slightly elevated left atrial pressure (pulmonary artery occlusion pressure <18 mmHg).

Acute lung injury (ALI) is the precursor to ARDS. Apart from a lesser degree of hypoxaemia (P_aO_2/F_iO_2 <300), the criteria for diagnosis are the same.

Epidemiology and prognosis

The **incidence** of ARDS is ~2–8 cases per 100 000 population per year, but its precursor ALI is much more common. ARDS mortality is generally **high (>50%)** but is determined by the precipitating condition (~35% for trauma, ~60% for sepsis and ~80% for aspiration pneumonia). Age (>60 years) and sepsis are also associated with increased mortality. Early diagnosis and treatment may improve outcome. The cause of death is **multiorgan failure (MOF)**, usually due to a combination of tissue hypoxia and overwhelming secondary infection. Less than 20% of patients die from hypoxaemia alone.

Pathogenesis (Fig. 40a) and causes (Fig. 40c)

During the **acute inflammatory phase** of ARDS, cytokine-activated neutrophils and monocytes adhere to pulmonary endothelium or alveolar epithelium, releasing inflammatory mediators and proteolytic enzymes (Chapter 18). These damage the integrity of the alveolar–capillary membrane, increase permeability and cause alveolar oedema. Reduced surfactant production causes alveolar collapse and hyaline membrane formation. The loss of functioning alveoli and ventilation/perfusion mismatch leads to progressive hypoxaemia and respiratory failure. The subsequent late **healing fibroproliferative phase** results in progressive pulmonary fibrosis and reduced compliance (stiff lungs). Associated pulmonary hypertension is partially due to activation of the coagulation cascade, with pulmonary capillary microthrombosis and regional hypoxic vasoconstriction.

Clinical features

The **acute inflammatory phase** lasts 3–10 days and results in hypoxaemia and MOF. It presents with progressive breathlessness, tachypnoea, central cyanosis, hypoxic confusion and lung crepitations. These symptoms and signs are in no way diagnostic and are shared with many other pulmonary conditions. During the later **healing, fibroproliferative phase**, pulmonary fibrosis (lung scarring) and pneumothoraces (Chapter 33) are common. Secondary chest and systemic infections complicate both phases.

Investigations

Monitoring: routine measurements include temperature, respiratory rate, O_2 saturation and urine output. In addition, the arterial and central venous pressures, the cardiac output and occasionally the left atrial pressure (using a pulmonary artery catheter) are measured **to assess fluid balance and ensure adequate tissue oxygen delivery**. Serial blood gas measurements are used to monitor gas exchange. Early detection of secondary pulmonary infection requires microbiological examination of sputum or bronchoalveolar lavage. **Radiological:** serial chest X-rays (CXRs) identify progression of **diffuse bilateral pulmonary infiltrates**. Similarly, early computed tomography (CT) scanning can identify **diffuse patchy infiltrates** with **dependent consolidation**; later scans reveal **pneumothoraces, pneumatoceles** and **fibrosis**.

Management

The key to successful management of ARDS is to **establish and treat the underlying cause**. In the early stages, oxygen therapy and physiotherapy may suffice. With progressive respiratory failure, non-invasive ventilation—with continuous positive airway pressure (CPAP) or non-invasive positive pressure ventilation (NIPPV)—or full mechanical ventilation and high-inspired oxygen concentrations may be required to maintain adequate ventilation and oxygenation. The high airways pressures needed to achieve normal tidal volumes during mechanical ventilation often result in lung damage (barotrauma), including pneumothorax and lung cysts. This ventilator-induced lung injury and oxygen toxicity ($F_iO_2 > 0.8$) must be prevented, as these contribute to mortality and multiorgan failure.

The basic principles of mechanical ventilation are to **limit pressure-induced damage, optimize oxygenation** and **avoid circulatory compromise** (reduced cardiac output and blood pressure due to high intrathoracic pressures; see also Chapter 41). A 'protective lung ventilation strategy' of low tidal volumes (6 mL/kg) and low peak inspiratory pressures (<30 cmH$_2$O) reduce lung damage, complications and mortality. **Alveolar recruitment** (of collapsed alveoli) is achieved with high positive end-expiratory pressures (PEEP >10 cmH$_2$O) or long inspiratory–expiratory times. The CO_2 retention ('permissive hypercapnia') resulting from this strategy of low tidal volume ventilation can be tolerated for long periods.

Excessive fluid loading must be avoided, as this increases the alveolar flooding characteristic of ARDS. The aim must be to maintain adequate perfusion of other organs while using the lowest possible left atrial pressures. In the acute situation, diuretics may be essential to correct hypoxaemia by reducing extravascular lung water. Thereafter, combinations of pulmonary and systemic vasodilators (before and after load reduction of the left heart), inotropes and vasoconstrictor agents may be used to achieve adequate cardiac output and perfusion pressures at low left atrial filling pressures.

Essential general measures include good nursing care, physiotherapy, nutrition and infection control. Reducing fever (shivering) and controlling anxiety with sedation decreases metabolic demand. **No drug therapy has been consistently beneficial** in early ARDS, including steroids, anti-inflammatory agents, anti-cytokines or surfactant therapy. However, 7–10 days after onset, steroid therapy may prevent the development of subsequent pulmonary fibrosis. **Inhaled nitric oxide** and nursing the patient in the **prone position** improves gas exchange by increasing perfusion to ventilated areas of lung, but no survival benefit has been demonstrated (Fig. 40d). **Extracorporeal membrane oxygenation (ECMO)** techniques to oxygenate blood or remove CO_2 are effective in children, but the benefit in adults has not been established.

41 Mechanical ventilation

(a) Indications for mechanical ventilation or support in adults

Surgery General anaesthesia with neuromuscular blockade Post operative management following major surgery	Cervical cord damage above C4 Neck fractures
Respiratory centre depression Usually when P_aCO_2 >7–8 kPa (50–60 mmHg) Head injury Drug overdose, e.g. opiates, barbiturates Raised intracranial pressure: cerebral haemorrhage/ tumours/meningitis/encephalitis Status epilepticus	Neuromuscular disorders – when VC <20–30 mL/kg Guillain–Barré Myasthenia gravis Poliomyelitis Polyneuritis
	Chest wall disorders Kyphoscoliosis Trauma: especially flail segment (multiple rib fractures → section of chest wall unattached)
Lung disease Pneumonia Acute respiratory distress syndrome (ARDS) Severe asthma attack Acute exacerbation of chronic obstructive pulmonary disease (COPD), cystic fibrosis Trauma–lung contusion Pulmonary oedema	Other Cardiac arrest Severe circulatory shock Resistant hypoxia in type 1 respiratory failure (reduces oxygen consumption)

(c) Airway pressure profiles in different types of ventilation

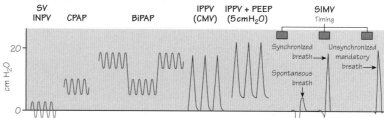

(b) Nasal mask and NIPPV

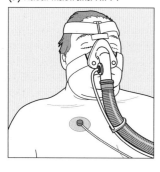

SV = spontaneous ventilation, INPV = intermittent negative pressure ventilation, CPAP = continuous positive airway pressure, BiPAP = biphasic continuous positive airway pressure, IPPV = intermittent positive pressure ventilation (= CMV), CMV = controlled mechanical ventilation, PEEP = positive end-expiratory pressure, SIMV = synchronized intermittent mandatory ventilation. If a spontaneous breath occurs in the timing window it triggers a synchronized ventilator breath and if not a mandatory breath is given soon after the timing window.

(d) Complications of mechanical ventilation

Risks during endotracheal intubation or tracheostomy Myocardial depression from anaesthetic Aspiration of gastric contents Fall in P_aO_2 during apnoea Reflex bronchoconstriction and laryngospasm	Risks associated with sedation and paralysis Cardiac depression Depression of respiratory drive (delays weaning) Increases danger of disconnection/ventilator failure
Risks of endotracheal intubation and tracheostomy Intubation of the oesophagus Intubation of a bronchus Blockage/accidental extubation Laryngeal/tracheal damage or stenosis Infection	Risks associated with mechanical ventilation High airway pressure → barotrauma Alveolar overdistension → volutrauma: • Pneumothorax, pneumomediastinum • Subcutaneous emphysema (= air in skin) • Structural damage to lung, airways and capillaries • Bronchopulmonary dysplasia (see Chapter 17)
Risks associated with high inspired oxygen (see Chapter 42)	

Mechanical ventilation is usually used to prevent or treat type 2 respiratory (ventilatory) failure. The main indications in adults are listed in Fig. 41a.

Types of mechanical ventilation (Fig. 41c)

Inspiratory muscle paralysis by poliomyelitis was a common reason for mechanical ventilation in the first half of the twentieth century. It was usually performed by **intermittent negative pressure ventilation (INPV)**, which is still occasionally used today. Patients are placed inside a **tank ventilator** sealed at the neck, and tank pressure is intermittently lowered, expanding the chest and lowering intrapleural pressure as in spontaneous breathing. Disadvantages of this **'iron lung'** include claustrophobia, discomfort, difficult nursing care and the bulk and expense of the equipment. **Jacket and cuirass ventilators** produce a negative pressure just around the chest, but difficulty in achieving a satisfactory seal limits their use to patients only needing ventilatory augmentation.

From the 1950s, **intermittent positive pressure ventilation (IPPV; controlled mechanical ventilation, CMV)** quickly replaced INPV for most purposes. Air is driven into the lungs by raising airway pressure, usually via an endotracheal or tracheostomy tube. Expiration is achieved by allowing pressure to fall to zero. This simple form of IPPV is used during routine surgery. Typical initial adult settings for IPPV are:

Tidal volume, $V_T = 8\text{--}12\,\text{mL/kg}$

Respiratory frequency, $f = 8\text{--}14\,\text{breaths/min}$

Minute ventilation, $V\ (= V_T \times f) \approx 6000\,\text{mL/min}$

Inspiratory time : expiratory time $= 1:2\text{--}1:3$

Minute ventilation is adjusted to maintain $P_a\text{CO}_2$ at about $5\,\text{kPa}$ ($37\,\text{mmHg}$). A slightly lower $P_a\text{CO}_2$ may be used initially in the presence of raised intracranial pressure. Accepting a higher $P_a\text{CO}_2$ (**permissive hypercapnia**) may prevent the need for excessively high airway pressures. $P_a\text{O}_2$ is maintained above $10\,\text{kPa}$ ($75\,\text{mmHg}$) by adjusting inspired $F\text{O}_2$. The lowest concentration needed is used, usually in the range 30–60%. It may be preferable to accept a slightly lower $P\text{O}_2$ than to use >60% for long periods.

Microprocessor control of ventilators has permitted development of numerous variations of IPPV. For example, in non-paralysed patients, the positive pressure may be synchronized with spontaneous breaths and a mandatory breath given if no spontaneous breaths occur in a preset time (**synchronized intermittent mandatory ventilation, SIMV**). In another form, the ventilator operates only where spontaneous ventilation falls below a preset minimum (**mandatory minute ventilation, MMV**).

If, instead of allowing airway pressure to fall to zero, a small positive pressure is maintained throughout expiration (**positive end-expiratory pressure, PEEP**), there is a reduction in V_A/Q mismatching and an improvement in $P_a\text{O}_2$ in some conditions, such as acute respiratory distress syndrome (ARDS). This occurs because PEEP increases functional residual capacity (FRC) and reduces the closure of airways and alveoli towards the end of expiration. Unfortunately,

intrathoracic pressure is raised, impairing venous return, and occasionally the fall in cardiac output can reduce tissue oxygen delivery despite the increased $P_a\text{O}_2$. The increased mean airway pressure caused by PEEP also increases the risk of barotrauma. A good compromise is to use the minimum PEEP required to keep $P\text{O}_2$ at an acceptable level (>$8\,\text{kPa}$, $60\,\text{mmHg}$) when breathing 50–60% oxygen.

Non-invasive respiratory support

Non-invasive ventilation avoids the use of tracheal intubation or tracheostomy. An example is INPV (above), but this is no longer widely used. In contrast, non-invasive positive pressure techniques using either a nasal mask (Fig. 41) or sometimes a full face mask are increasingly being used.

In **continuous positive airway pressure (CPAP)**, a standing pressure of 5–10 cmH$_2$O is applied to a nasal or face mask in a spontaneously breathing patient (Fig. 41c). This has several potential beneficial effects. First, it helps prevent upper airway collapse in **obstructive sleep apnoea**. In interstitial diseases such as **ARDS**, it recruits alveoli, reducing V_A/Q mismatching. FRC is increased, and this may increase lung compliance by moving the patient onto the steep part of the pressure–volume curve (Chapter 6). CO_2 retention may be a problem during CPAP, which may be improved by using biphasic or bilevel positive pressure ventilation (BiPAP). BiPAP alternates between high and low pressure either for fixed time periods (Fig. 41c) or between inspiration and expiration, improving the emptying of the lungs.

CPAP may improve oxygenation and may aid the patient's own respiratory efforts, but it cannot produce ventilation by itself. In contrast, **non-invasive intermittent positive pressure ventilation (NIPPV)** is IPPV delivered by face or, more usually, nasal mask. For it to be used successfully, the patient must be cooperative and introduced to the technique gradually, to allow synchronization of his or her breathing with the ventilator. Its use includes nocturnal ventilation of patients with chronic respiratory failure due to neuromuscular disease or thoracic deformity. It is being used increasingly to treat acute exacerbations of chronic obstructive pulmonary disease (COPD), avoiding the need for intubation and improving survival.

In summary, the main beneficial effect of **CPAP** is recruitment of alveoli. The reduction in collapse sometimes also gives rise to a reduction in the work of breathing. In contrast, **NIPPV** is used to reduce the work of breathing rather than to recruit alveoli. This may be of benefit in the tired (e.g. COPD) patient.

Weaning the patient off the ventilator following surgery is usually achieved by reversing neuromuscular blockade and lightening the anaesthetic level. In ICU patients, weaning may be more difficult. Several techniques are used, including removing mechanical ventilation for progressively longer periods, or by using a spontaneously breathing mode (e.g. SIMV), and pressure support in which support is progressively reduced. CPAP applied via the endotracheal tube may also help the weaning process.

Problems are hard to predict accurately, but are most likely following prolonged ventilation, in debilitated patients, or in those with neuromuscular or chronic respiratory disease. A pattern of rapid shallow breathing 5 minutes after disconnection from the ventilator is one of the more useful predictors of failure.

Complications of mechanical ventilation are numerous, and are listed in Fig. 41d.

Oxygen delivery systems

High-flow (Venturi) face mask

- The O_2 flow through the jet mixing Venturi valves draws the correct proportion of oxygen to produce the required O_2 concentration
- Delivers more mixed gas to the mask than the patient needs (e.g. 30 L/min)
- Inspired O_2 concentration unaffected by patient's breathing pattern
- Safest in COPD patients in respiratory failure

High-flow (Venturi) face mask

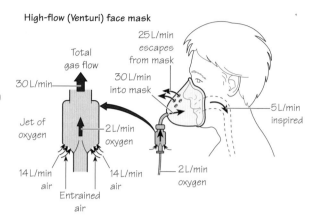

Low-flow masks

- Oxygen flows at a set rate into the mask and is supplemented by air drawn into the mask
- FiO_2 achieved depends on ventilation:

  Ventilation = 5 L/min

  Oxygen flow = 2 L/min   Air (21% O_2) = 3 L/min

  $FiO_2 = (2 + 0.21 \times 3) / 5 \times 100 = $ **53%**

  Ventilation = 25 L/min

  Oxygen flow = 2 L/min   Air (21% O_2) = 23 L/min

  $FiO_2 = (2 + 0.21 \times 23) / 25 \times 100 = $ **27%**

- Not recommended where accurate control of FiO_2 desirable, e.g. patients with COPD and chronic hypercapnia

Low-flow face mask

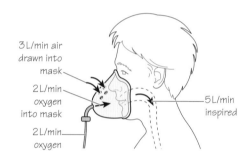

Nasal prongs

- Delivers a constant oxygen flow therefore PiO_2 varies with ventilation
- More comfortable than mask
- No need to remove to expectorate or eat
- O_2 delivered by nose is probably inhaled even in mouth breathing

Rebreathing and anaesthetic mask

- High concentration oxygen mask ($FiO_2 > 60\%$)
- Incorporate a degree of rebreathing ∴ risk of CO_2 retention

With non-invasive ventilation: may help where oxygen supplementation alone is not enough (see Chapter 41)

Nasal prongs

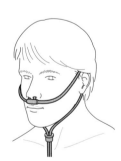

Correctly administered oxygen therapy can be life-saving. The wrong concentration and inadequate monitoring can have severe consequences.

Pathophysiology

Tissues require oxygen for survival. Oxygen utilization is dependent on delivery by the circulation of blood containing adequate quantities of oxygen in a readily releasable form to tissues capable of using the delivered oxygen. **Tissue hypoxia** can be caused by: **low arterial Po_2** (hypoxaemia); inadequate **tissue blood flow** (cardiac failure, emboli); low **haemoglobin concentration** (anaemia); abnormal **oxygen dissociation curve** (haemoglobinopathies, CO poisoning); and **poisoning of intracellular oxygen usage** (e.g. cyanide, sepsis). Tissue hypoxia occurs **within 4 minutes** of failure of any of these systems, because tissue and lung oxygen reserves are small. Successful treatment requires early recognition, but the clinical features are often non-specific, including altered mental state, dyspnoea, hyperventilation, arrhythmias and hypotension (for details, see Chapter 22). The effects of anaemia and abnormal dissociation curves are discussed in Chapter 8.

Measuring tissue hypoxia

Arterial oxygen saturation (S_aO_2) is measured with a **pulse oximeter**, and partial pressure of oxygen (P_aO_2) by **blood gas analysis**. These are the principal clinical measurements used for initiating, monitoring and adjusting oxygen therapy. However, these measures can be normal when tissue hypoxia is caused by low cardiac output states, anaemia and failure of tissue oxygen use. In these circumstances, **mixed venous oxygen partial pressure** (P_vO_2), which is measured in blood taken from a pulmonary artery catheter, approximates to mean tissue Po_2. Severe hypoxia in a single organ (e.g. due to an arterial embolus) may be associated with a normal P_aO_2, S_aO_2 and P_vO_2. Measurement of individual organ hypoxia is difficult, and requires specialized techniques (e.g. tonometry).

Acute oxygen therapy

The main indications for instituting oxygen therapy are:
Hypoxaemia ($P_aO_2 < 7.8$ kPa, $S_aO_2 < 90\%$).
Hypotension (systolic blood pressure < 100 mmHg).
Low cardiac output and metabolic acidosis (bicarbonate < 18 mmol/L).
Respiratory distress (respiratory rate > 24/min).
The airway should be checked before starting oxygen therapy, and arterial blood gases analysed as soon as possible to assess P_aO_2, P_aCO_2, pH and bicarbonate.

In the acute situation, the **dose of oxygen may be critical**. Inadequate oxygen accounts for more death and disability than can be justified by the small risks associated with high-dose oxygen. Short periods of high-dose oxygen may preserve life until more specific therapy (e.g. antibiotics, thrombolytics) can be instituted. When blood gas results are available, the dose of oxygen can be adjusted to maintain the P_aO_2 between 8 and 10 kPa. The recommended initial oxygen concentrations as a fraction of oxygen in inspired air (F_iO_2 in percentage) are:
Cardiac or respiratory arrest, 100%.
Hypoxaemia with $P_aCO_2 < 5.3$ kPa, 40–60%.
Hypoxaemia with $P_aCO_2 > 5.3$ kPa, initially 24%.
The important features, advantages and disadvantages of different **oxygen delivery systems** are shown in Fig. 42.

Dangers of oxygen therapy

Carbon dioxide retention: high-dose oxygen given to the 10–15% of chronic obstructive pulmonary disease (COPD) patients with type 2 respiratory failure (Chapter 22) will reduce hypoxic drive to breath, increase V/Q mismatching, and may cause CO_2 retention and respiratory acidosis that may be lethal. Fortunately, as these patients are on the steep part of the oxygen dissociation curve, small increases in P_aO_2 cause worthwhile improvements in arterial oxygen content. The initial oxygen concentration should be low (24–28%) and progressively increased if repeat blood gas analysis shows little or no increase in P_aCO_2. The aim is to correct hypoxaemia ($P_aO_2 > 6.65$ kPa) without decreasing arterial pH below 7.26. Non-invasive positive pressure ventilation and respiratory stimulants may improve ventilation and prevent CO_2 retention. **Pulmonary oxygen toxicity:** $F_iO_2 > 60\%$ may damage the alveolar membrane if inhaled for >24–48 h. **Fire:** facial burns and deaths occur when patients smoke while using oxygen. **Absorption collapse:** if an airway becomes blocked, oxygen in the trapped alveolar gas is rapidly absorbed, but N_2 absorption is slow, as alveolar P_{N_2} is in equilibrium with mixed venous P_{N_2}. If N_2 is replaced by O_2 during oxygen therapy, temporary blockage of airways by secretions is more likely to lead to collapsed alveoli, which may be difficult to reopen.

Efficacy of acute oxygen therapy

Arterial hypoxaemia

Right-to-left shunting (e.g. pneumonic consolidation): when shunt is >20%, hypoxia persists despite high F_iO_2 (Chapter 13).

Alveolar hypoventilation (e.g. drug overdose, neuromuscular disorders): oxygen rapidly corrects hypoxaemia, but the high P_aCO_2 remains. The primary aim is to improve ventilation.

V/Q mismatch (in COPD or asthma, Chapter 14): improved oxygenation, but the response will vary between patients.

Tissue hypoxia without arterial hypoxaemia

Low-output cardiac states (congestive cardiac failure, CCF; myocardial infarction, MI): oxygen solubility is low, and even at F_iO_2 100%, only 30% of total oxygen requirement is carried dissolved in blood. In the absence of hypoxaemia, high oxygen can only marginally improve tissue oxygenation by a small increase in dissolved oxygen. This may preserve some cells with critical oxygen supply, but it must not delay correction of the primary clinical problem (e.g. restoring tissue blood flow).

Chronic lung disease: relief of breathlessness is reported in some patients without hypoxaemia, and a trial of oxygen may be warranted.

Carbon monoxide poisoning: a high F_iO_2 is essential despite a normal P_aO_2, because oxygen competes for haemoglobin binding sites and reduces the half-life of carboxyhaemoglobin from about 320 to 80 minutes.

Monitoring oxygen therapy

Careful monitoring of oxygen therapy by oximetry (S_aO_2) and arterial blood gas measurement is essential. Oximetry has the advantage of continuous oxygen measurement, whereas blood gases are required to monitor P_aCO_2 and pH.

Stopping oxygen therapy

Oxygen therapy should be stopped when the arterial oxygenation is adequate with the patient breathing room air ($P_aO_2 > 8$ kPa, $S_aO_2 > 90\%$). In patients without arterial hypoxaemia, oxygen should be stopped when the acid–base state and clinical assessment are consistent with resolution of tissue hypoxia.

43 Sleep-disordered breathing

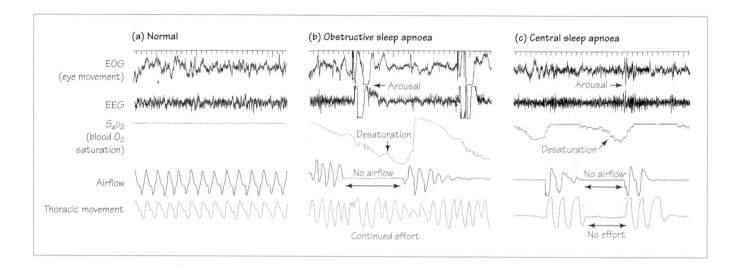

(a) Normal | (b) Obstructive sleep apnoea | (c) Central sleep apnoea

EOG (eye movement)
EEG
S_aO_2 (blood O_2 saturation)
Airflow
Thoracic movement

Arousal — Desaturation — No airflow — Continued effort (b)

Arousal → Desaturation — No airflow — No effort (c)

Sleep-disordered breathing is common, with a vast potential for improvement in quality of life. Normal sleep (Fig. 43) consists of rapid eye movement (**REM**, ~25%) and non-rapid eye movement (**NREM**) sleep. REM sleep is characterized by an awake-pattern electroencephalography (EEG), voluntary muscle atonia and dreaming. Ventilatory drive is normally diminished in REM sleep, causing a slight fall in P_aO_2 and a rise in P_aCO_2. Daytime hypersomnolence due to sleep deprivation and sleep fragmentation may lead to decreased quality of life, including increased risk of accidents and cognitive dysfunction. It may be due to a variety of causes, including **obstructive sleep apnoea** and more rarely **central sleep apnoea**. Sleep-disordered breathing is diagnosed using **polysomnography** (Fig. 43), which records the EEG for sleep patterns, movements of abdomen and thorax to assess breathing, oronasal flow and oximetry for O_2 saturation.

Obstructive sleep apnoea (OSA) is characterized by absence of airflow with continued respiratory effort (Fig. 43b). About 90% of patients with sleep apnoea have OSA. OSA is far more common in males than females, and is associated with alcohol consumption, increasing age, obesity, increased neck circumference, hypertension and hypothyroidism. Obstruction typically occurs in the upper airway and pharynx, and is related to the normal decreases in upper airway muscle tone and increased airway resistance that occur in REM sleep. These factors, in conjunction with individual anatomy and posture, result in airway collapse during inspiration, when airway pressure is reduced. Apnoea resolves with arousal and restoration of muscle tone. Although hundreds or thousands of episodes of apnoea and arousal may occur each night, patients are often unaware of them; sleep partners commonly report **loud snoring**, snorting or apnoea. Patients develop **daytime hypersomnolence** and **gain weight**, and may show pedal oedema, nasal congestion, enlarged tongue, shallow palate, enlarged uvula or retrognathia. Most patients have normal arterial blood gases and haemoglobin. In chronic obstructive pulmonary disease (COPD), **nocturnal hypoxia** can be severe even with mild OSA, as gas exchange is already compromised.

Polysomnography reveals repeated episodes of OSA or hypopnoea (reduced airflow with oxygen desaturation or arousal), which terminate with arousal (Fig. 43b). These episodes are quantified by the **apnoea plus hypopnoea index** (**AHI**, episodes/h). Normal sleep has an AHI < 10. Severe OSA usually has an AHI > 40. A minority of patients with very severe OSA may develop **obesity hypoventilation syndrome** (Pickwick syndrome). Obstructive episodes can cause **pulmonary hypertension** (Chapter 26) from hypoxic pulmonary vasoconstriction. Systemic blood pressure increases during apnoea, possibly due to sympathetic stimulation, and left ventricle (LV) afterload increases during obstructive apnoeas due to the marked fall in pleural pressure. There is a strong association between OSA and systemic hypertension, although the cause is unknown.

Therapy requires relief of obstruction. Moderate weight loss (≥10%) often results in substantial improvements. **Nasal continuous positive airway pressure** (**CPAP**, Chapter 41) is the most commonly prescribed therapy, but 50% of patients do not comply in the long-term. Some patients respond to oral appliances or uvulopalatopharyngoplasty (surgery). O_2 alone may decrease or eliminate hypoxia, but not the obstruction or arousals.

Central sleep apnoea (CSA) is characterized by cessation of airflow during sleep without evidence of respiratory effort, and is due to a **loss or inhibition of central respiratory drive** (Fig. 43c). Patients with CSA may be subdivided into those with daytime hypercapnia or normocapnia. CSA with daytime hypercapnia is usually due to central alveolar hypoventilation, neuromuscular disease or chest wall disease (e.g. kyphoscoliosis). Central alveolar hypoventilation may be primary (Ondine's curse) or secondary to brainstem disease (Chapter 12). Neuromuscular causes include muscular dystrophy, phrenic nerve dysfunction, myositis (muscle inflammation) and myasthenia gravis. Patients with a CNS cause for hypoventilation ('won't breathe') may benefit from a respiratory stimulant. Patients with weakness or chest wall disease ('can't breathe') benefit from assisted mechanical ventilation (Chapter 41).

44 Case studies: questions

Case 1: Pulmonary emboli

At the start of your shift on an orthopaedic ward you are asked to review two patients.

Elizabeth is a 70-year-old who was making a good recovery from her hip replacement 3 days ago. This morning while eating breakfast she developed sudden breathlessness. She denies any pain.

Alice is a 35-year-old woman who had an internal fixation of a femoral shaft fracture following a road traffic accident 4 days earlier. This morning she complains of pleuritic pain but no breathlessness.

Initial clinical findings for Elizabeth are: blood pressure (BP) of 110/80 mmHg, heart rate (HR) 95 beats/min, respiratory rate 24 breaths/min and oxygen saturation 86%. Initial clinical findings for Alice are: BP 126/80 mmHg, HR 80 beats/min, respiratory rate 18 breaths/min and oxygen saturation 97%.

In both patients, examination is otherwise unremarkable and the initial chest X-ray and electrocardiogram (ECG) are normal, although a repeat X-ray the following day shows that Alice has developed a small right-sided pleural effusion.

Questions

1 You are worried whether either or both could have a pulmonary embolus (PE). From the history and findings so far is this likely in either or both of these patients? If these patients had not had surgery recently but had presented with the same symptoms and signs in Accident and Emergency, would your answer be different?

2 Which of these oxygen saturations is 'typical' of a pulmonary embolus?

3 Pulmonary emboli produce an area of lung that is ventilated but not perfused, that is they produce alveolar dead space and therefore increase physiological dead space. Does increased physiological dead space inevitably lead to a reduced arterial P_{O_2}?

4 What other aspects of the history might be relevant?

5 D-dimer tests are a useful addition to the diagnostic armoury but false positives are common. False negatives also occur. Which sort of PE is most likely to be associated with a false negative PE? How long do D-dimers remain elevated?

6 What is the role of CXR and ECG? How will they be affected in the presence of a pulmonary embolus?

7 What other investigations are appropriate?

8 What are the treatment options for Elizabeth and Alice?

Case 2: Asthma

Tom, who is 15 years old, attends his GP's asthma clinic. He has had asthma since early childhood. On two occasions, when he was 8 and 10 years old, he had attacks severe enough to require hospital admission. At present, his asthma is well controlled on regular inhaled beclometasone dipropionate 200 μg twice daily and inhaled salmeterol 50 μg twice daily. Today, his peak flow is 510 L/min (predicted value for his age and height 530 L/min). On auscultation, there is vesicular breathing and no other sounds.

Questions

1 Is this peak flow normal? Apart from the nomogram values, can you think of any other peak flow reading with which it would be useful to compare today's clinic reading?

2 If you measured the following:
- FEV_1/FVC
- Airway resistance
- Functional residual capacity (FRC)
- Lung compliance
- Arterial P_{O_2} and arterial P_{CO_2}

—how would they compare with the normal for a boy of his age and size?

On a school trip to a countryside park, Tom becomes breathless running across a field. His teacher is alarmed by his noisy breathing and asks you, a passing medical student, to assess whether they need to get him to hospital.

3 What simple observations can you make that will help you decide how severe this attack is? In his backpack he has a salbutamol inhaler, a salmeterol inhaler, a sodium cromoglycate inhaler and a beclometasone inhaler. Which should he use?

4 If you had been able to measure the following during his episode of breathlessness:
- FEV_1/FVC
- Peak flow rate
- Airway resistance
- Functional residual capacity
- Lung compliance
- Arterial P_{O_2} and arterial P_{CO_2}

—how do you think they would compare with the normal for a boy of his age and size?

5 If you had had your stethoscope with you, what would you have heard on examining his chest?

At 18 years of age, Tom goes to college in London. He stops taking regular medication, as he feels he has 'grown out' of his asthma. He keeps a salbutamol inhaler in his room 'just in case'. During the first term he is well, apart from a couple of wheezy episodes while playing football. In the second term, he develops a heavy cold, and over 24 h he becomes progressively more breathless despite frequent puffs of salbutamol. His friends call out his GP, who finds the following: Tom is fully alert, but talking in broken sentences because he is very breathless. He is not cyanosed. He is using his accessory muscles of respiration. On auscultation, there are widespread expiratory rhonchi (wheezes). BP is 115/80 mmHg, HR 110 beats/min, respiratory rate 30 breaths/min, peak flow 200 L/min.

6 Which observations suggest that this is a fairly severe attack?

7 If the GP had measured airway resistance, FRC, lung compliance, arterial P_{O_2} and P_{CO_2}, how would they compare to the predicted values?

His GP decides that this attack warrants hospital admission, and he calls an ambulance. Unfortunately, owing to heavy traffic it is 40 min before he arrives at the local Accident and Emergency department. By this time, Tom is confused, too breathless to talk and unable to produce a peak flow reading. The Accident and Emergency officer notices he is now cyanosed, although the widespread rhonchi noted in the GP's letter have now disappeared. Arterial blood gases show arterial P_{O_2} = 7 kPa and arterial P_{CO_2} = 5.5 kPa while breathing 60% oxygen.

8 Discuss the features that suggest this asthma attack is life-threatening. Do the reduced rhonchi on auscultation contradict the other findings?

9 What is the cause of the low arterial P_{O_2}? Was the inhaled oxygen helpful, and if so was the correct concentration used? Is this P_{CO_2} normal, and how does it affect your assessment of the severity of this attack?

Case 3: Severe breathlessness

A 38-year-old man is seen for evaluation of severe exertional dyspnoea. Two years ago, he had been able to play squash regularly, but he stopped 6 months ago because of dyspnoea and fatigue during exercise. He now reports dyspnoea after climbing one flight of stairs. He has no cough, sputum or wheeze. He smoked one pack of cigarettes a day for 10 years and quit 7 years ago. He has no allergies or pets, and has not travelled outside of Europe or the USA. One of his six siblings died at age 25 with an unknown progressive lung ailment.

Physical examination was notable for a thin male, BP was 110/75 mmHg, HR was 104, respiratory rate was 22, oxygen saturation 96% at rest; chest with diminished breath sounds and a prolonged expiratory phase, slightly elevated jugular venous pressure, scaphoid abdomen, no hepatomegaly, but with a trace of pedal oedema. His haematocrit was 45% and other laboratory tests were normal.

Chest radiograph shows flat diaphragm with increased radiolucency at the lung bases.

Lung function tests	Measured	% Predicted
FEV$_1$ (L)	0.80	20
FVC (L)	3.0	60
FEV$_1$/FVC	0.27	33
TLC (L)	8.1	120
D_LCO (mL/min/mmHg)	14	45

Questions

1 What would you expect the patient's FRC and residual volume (RV) to be?
2 Why is the cardiac PMI shifted to the midline?
3 Why is the FVC low?
4 Why is the D_LCO low?
5 What will happen to the patient's oxygenation with exercise? Why?
6 Why is the patient's jugular venous pressure elevated?
7 What are the most likely diagnosis and pathophysiology of his disease?

Case 4: Restrictive ventilatory defect

Two 60-year-old patients are being evaluated for dyspnoea. On examination, both patients have an oxygen saturation of 88%, small lung volumes to percussion and normal cardiac examinations. Patient A has diffuse bilateral

Lung function tests	Patient A		Patient B	
	Measured	% Predicted	Measured	% Predicted
FEV$_1$ (L)	1.1	26	1.1	26
FVC (L)	1.3	26	1.3	26
FEV$_1$/FVC	0.80	100	0.80	100
TLC (L)	3.0	43	3.8	54
FRC (L)	2.0	54	3.1	87
RV (L)	1.7	65	2.5	120
D_LCO (mL/min/mmHg)	18	50	36	100

inspiratory crackles and digital clubbing. Patient B has clear lungs and difficulty in rising from his chair and raising his hands over his head.

Questions

1 What patterns of abnormalities do these patients exhibit?
2 Based on the lung function results, what is the most likely pathophysiology explaining each patient's symptoms?
3 What is the likely explanation for the differences in FRC and RV between the two patients?
4 What is the differential diagnosis for Patient A?
5 What is the differential diagnosis for Patient B?
6 Both patients have hypoxemia. Which patient is more likely to have hypercapnia?

Case 5: Haemoptysis

A 31-year-old married Vietnamese woman presented to the Accident and Emergency department following an episode of haemoptysis in which she had expectorated 250 mL fresh red blood. Nasopharyngeal examination by the ENT surgeons was normal, and a chest radiograph (Fig. 44) in the Accident and Emergency department was unhelpful, although bronchial wall thickening was noted behind the heart (arrow). There was no further bleeding, and she was discharged with an outpatient appointment. Over the next few days, she continued to expectorate small clots of blood mixed with discolored phlegm.

At her outpatient appointment, she reported a 10-year history of recurrent, intermittent haemoptysis in which she had expectorated small quantities of fresh red blood, sometimes mixed with bronchial secretions. She had been investigated by several doctors, but chest radiographs were normal, and she had been reassured that the bleeding was from the upper respiratory tract. For the 6 months before her presentation to the Accident and Emergency department, she had coughed up small quantities of blood every 2–3 weeks (<50 mL), but there was no associated fever, wheeze or breathlessness on these occasions. Two weeks before presentation to the Accident and Emergency department, she developed a cough productive of purulent sputum and night-time sweating. As a child, she had suffered with whooping cough, but there was no other past medical history of serious chest illness or tuberculosis. She is a non-smoker.

Examination was normal. She did not have finger clubbing, anaemia, cyanosis or lymphadenopathy. Chest examination was unremarkable. The breath sounds were vesicular, and there were no crackles or

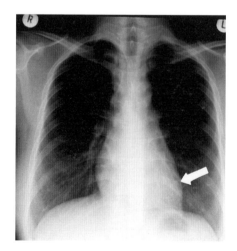

Fig. 44 Chest radiograph.

wheezes. Routine blood tests, including an erythrocyte sedimentation rate (ESR) and C-reactive protein and sputum microbiology including examination for tuberculosis, were normal. The grade 1 Heaf test was consistent with immunity to tuberculosis.

Questions

1 What are the most common causes of haemoptysis, and from which circulation does bleeding occur?

2 Is haemoptysis life-threatening, and how is the severity of bleeding classified?

3 What are the clinical features that may help establish the diagnosis? What is the most likely cause in this case?

4 What investigations would you perform to establish the diagnosis in this case?

5 What is bronchiectasis, and what causes it?

6 How should a large haemoptysis be managed?

Case 1: Pulmonary emboli

1 Pulmonary embolism can be asymptomatic or present with a variety of different symptoms and signs including sudden death. Breathlessness and pain, which is typically pleuritic, are the most common symptoms followed by cough. Haemoptysis is relatively uncommon occurring in only about one in six patients. Other presentations and symptoms include hypotension and syncope, wheezing, and sudden onset of atrial fibrillation. Symptoms and signs of a deep venous thrombosis (DVT), such as swelling and pain in the calf may also be present but they are often absent. Both these patients have had recent orthopaedic surgery and are in a high risk group for DVT and pulmonary embolus. In this context sudden onset of breathlessness and/or pleuritic pain makes pulmonary embolism a serious possibility. In patients without a history of recent surgery or fracture presenting in an Accident and Emergency department with recent onset of breathlessness or pleuritic pain, pulmonary embolus would be a less likely explanation for these symptoms but still a real possibility even in those with no other recognized risk factors (see answer 3).

2 Either of these oxygen saturations is entirely compatible with the diagnosis of pulmonary embolus. A low P_aO_2 and arterial oxygen saturation is common especially with the larger, more proximally lodged emboli, whereas oxygen saturation may be normal with smaller emboli that lodge more peripherally.

3 No, with a moderately increased physiological dead space hypoxia can be avoided if the subject increases respiratory rate and/or tidal volume sufficiently to compensate for the increased dead space ventilation, restoring alveolar ventilation to its previous level. However, pulmonary embolism leads to other problems such as reduced surfactant production, areas of atelectasis and increased ventilation–perfusion mismatching. The effects of ventilation–perfusion mismatching may be made worse by decreased mixed venous oxygen content resulting from a reduced cardiac output. As a result, hypoxia and an increased A–a P_{O_2} gradient are common with pulmonary emboli. As expected with ventilation–perfusion mismatching, P_aCO_2 is usually reduced.

4 Other risk factors may be revealed. These include pregnancy, oestrogen therapy, cancer, malignancy, chemotherapy, previous DVT, myocardial infarction, inflammatory bowel disease, immobolization or recent long distance travel. A previous or family history of venous thrombosis will suggest an inherited problem with the coagulation system such as Factor V Leiden. On examination a raised jugular venous pressure and/or a pleural rub would increase suspicion.

5 D-dimers are fibrin degradation products. They are not specific to pulmonary embolus or DVT but may be raised in sepsis, trauma (including surgery) and malignancy so false positives are common. With the most sensitive assays false negatives are less common but may occur with small peripheral emboli. Following a pulmonary embolus they remain elevated for about 6 days following the onset of symptoms. In the clinical context of low probability of pulmonary embolus negative D-dimers can be the end of the investigation. If D-dimers are positive or clinical probability high then further investigation is likely to be appropriate.

Small peripheral emboli may also be missed by other techniques such as computed tomography pulmonary angiogram (CTPA). They tend to cause pleuritic pain but less breathlessness and haemodynamic disturbance than larger emboli, which lodge in more proximal pulmonary arteries. There is some controversy about whether failing to detect such emboli matters. They are likely to clear without treatment but on the other hand they may herald further, more significant emboli.

6 Both the chest X-ray (CXR) and the electrocardiogram (ECG) may show abnormalities but none of the abnormalities are specific to pulmonary emboli. In the presence of a pulmonary embolus the X-ray may be normal initially but abnormalities such as areas of atelectasis, parenchymal densities and pleural effusions often develop over the first day or so. Pleural effusions are usually small, often bloody and resolve over a few days. An increasing pleural effusion suggests another cause for the symptoms or recurrent emboli. The ECG may be completely normal or show non-specific changes. Other changes that may be found are associated with right ventricular strain such as the S1, Q3, T3 pattern (prominent S wave in lead I, Q wave and inverted T in lead III), right axis deviation, dominant R wave in lead V1, inverted T waves in leads V1–V3 and right bundle branch block.

Probably the most important role of the CXR and ECG is to reveal alternative causes of symptoms such as dyspnoea and chest pain, such as pneumothorax or myocardial infarction.

7 Diagnosing pulmonary emboli is difficult and as yet there is no single test that is highly sensitive, highly specific, non-invasive, readily available and suitable for all situations. Various algorithms and investigation strategies have been proposed that take into account risk factors and the clinical situation but this still remains a difficult area with problems of both under- and over-diagnosis. Radionucleide ventilation–perfusion scans, spiral/helical computed tomography (CTPA) and pulmonary angiograms all have advantages and disadvantages which are discussed in Chapter 27. Demonstrating a DVT using Doppler imaging or venography is helpful, both because it greatly increases the likelihood that pulmonary symptoms are embolic in origin and also because the treatment is the same for both.

8 Anticoagulation with heparin and then warfarin for 6 months is the standard treatment for proven pulmonary emboli (see Chapter 27) but for Elizabeth and Alice this option is complicated by their recent surgery which would increase the risk of haemorrhagic complications. An inferior vena cava filter is an alternative and may be necessary to prevent further fatal emboli. This is a further reason why vigorous prophylaxis (see Chapter 27) is essential in high-risk patients. Thrombolysis is sometimes considered in large emboli with haemodynamic effects but would be contraindicated here by the recent surgery.

Case 2: Asthma

1 For males, peak flow should be no more than 100 L/min below the predicted; Tom's peak flow is therefore within the normal range for his age and size. The most useful value to compare it with would be his own best peak flow rate.

2 All of these should be normal. Asthma, especially in the young, is reversible, and between attacks patients usually have normal airway resistance, compliance, lung volumes and blood gases. Peak flow and auscultation (but see note in answer 9) suggest little evidence of airway obstruction today.

3 Simple observations that can be made in these circumstances are as follow:

- How breathless is he? Inability to talk in complete sentences is an indication of a severe attack.

- Respiratory rate (>25 breaths/min suggests a severe attack).
- Cyanosis (very severe attack).
- Pulse rate (>110 beats/min suggests a severe attack).
- If he has his peak flow meter with him a value <50% of his best or predicted suggests severe attack.

Even in the absence of the above signs of a severe attack, it is important to monitor the response to treatment to ensure that improvement rather than deterioration is occurring. He should use a short-acting β_2-adrenoreceptor agonist (salbutamol), which relaxes bronchial smooth muscle (see Chapter 24).

4 He now has definite bronchoconstriction; we would expect both peak flow and FEV_1/FVC to be reduced. In this mild attack, he would probably be able to exhale completely, so functional residual capacity (FRC) is likely to be normal. There is at present no reason why lung compliance should be altered. Although he will be working harder than normal, he should be achieving a normal alveolar ventilation and his blood gases should be normal. A reduced arterial P_{CO_2} may be caused by anxiety and consequent hyperventilation.

5 Expiratory rhonchi (musical sounds caused by vibration of the sides of collapsing airways).

6 The broken sentences, use of accessory muscles, high heart and respiratory rate are all important. The peak flow is only about 40% of his best value.

7 This is clearly a severe asthma attack, and airway resistance would be greatly increased. It is likely that air trapping would occur, as initially expiration is affected more than inspiration. As expiration is slowed, the subject may be forced to breathe in before the last breath has been fully exhaled, or air may be trapped behind collapsed airways. This would lead to a raised FRC. The volume–pressure curve flattens as total lung capacity (TLC) is approached (i.e. compliance is reduced). Consequently, with this severity of attack, the work of breathing is increased not only because of increased work against airway resistance, but also because of increased elastic resistance. In addition, with increased FRC, the inspiratory muscles may not be at their optimum working length and hence efficiency is impaired. Some ventilation–perfusion mismatching would be expected, as bronchoconstriction and inflammation will result in under-ventilation of some regions, and with the resulting shunt effect there is likely to be some degree of arterial hypoxia. Increased total ventilation will usually lower the P_{CO_2}, resulting in a final blood gas picture of low P_{O_2} and low P_{CO_2}.

8 The cyanosis indicates severe hypoxia, and is probably responsible for his confused mental state. The inability to talk and produce a peak flow reading are also signs of life-threatening asthma. The disappearance of rhonchi is consistent with very poor air movement. Rhonchi are a characteristic feature of airway obstruction, but they are not a reliable indicator of severity. In life-threatening asthma, the normal vesicular breath sounds are also absent. A silent chest in an asthma attack is an ominous sign.

9 The low P_aO_2 is caused by ventilation–perfusion mismatching. Hypoxia is what kills in severe asthma, so it is appropriate to give high inspired oxygen, which should significantly raise alveolar oxygen tension in poorly ventilated regions of his lung, and so improve arterial oxygenation. In this patient, there is no need to worry about ventilatory drive, so as high as possible is the correct emergency treatment. With a face mask, the maximum achievable is ~60%. Although a P_{CO_2} of 5.5 kPa would usually be considered 'normal', in the presence of severe hypoxia it should be regarded as worrying. With this degree of hypoxia, the drive to breathing should be increased, with increased ventilation and low P_{CO_2}. Here the failure to raise ventilation appropriately is

likely to indicate exhaustion. The patient may deteriorate rapidly—a further fall in ventilation will worsen hypoxia, and this may be fatal. In the presence of significant hypoxia, a 'normal' or high arterial P_{CO_2} should be regarded as a serious finding.

Case 3: Severe breathlessness

1 The obstructive ventilatory defect (low ratio of FEV_1/FVC) coupled with a reduced diffusing capacity for carbon monoxide would suggest emphysema. Emphysema is characterized by a reduction in lung elastic recoil, increased lung compliance and floppy airways. Therefore, FRC and residual volume (RV) are both likely to be elevated.

2 The hyperinflation of the lung and the increase in FRC pulls the apex of the heart caudally and to the middle. This can be seen radiographically as a small midline heart. The ECG will show low voltage due to the increased amount of air between the heart and the chest wall, with an axis close to 90°. For a similar reason, the apex beat may be quiet.

3 The forced vital capacity (FVC) is low because the RV is high. Airways close prematurely in emphysema, which increases RV. Furthermore, because of the marked decrease in maximal expiratory flow rate due to the decreased lung elastic recoil, patients' spirometry traces may not plateau, indicating that the lung was still emptying at very low flow rates when the FVC manoeuvre was terminated.

4 Diffusing capacity is influenced by the alveolar–capillary surface area for gas exchange. Emphysema is characterized by a loss of the alveolar–capillary units that are utilized for diffusion. There need not be a defect in transfer of gas from the alveolus to the capillary to reduce the D_{LCO}; a reduction in surface area is adequate to cause abnormality.

5 With exercise, the patient's oxygen saturation will fall because of the diffusion defect. With this magnitude of diffusion defect, the red cells have adequate time to equilibrate with alveolar oxygen as they traverse the alveolar–capillary membrane. However, during exercise, when cardiac output rises, red cells traverse the alveolar–capillary membrane at rest more quickly and do not equilibrate with alveolar oxygen tension at the end-capillary segment. This results in deoxygenated blood entering the systemic circulation when cardiac output is increased. This exercise-induced desaturation will be accentuated when alveolar oxygen is reduced, such as at high altitude. The threshold for significant oxygen desaturation with exercise is approximately D_{LCO} <50% predicted.

6 The patient probably has a component of pulmonary hypertension due to the emphysema. The loss of capillary units raises pulmonary vascular resistance and increases right heart work. Any degree of hypoxaemia during exercise will exacerbate the pulmonary hypertension by superimposing hypoxic pulmonary vasoconstriction on the already increased resistance.

7 The presence of early onset emphysema, the family history and the history of cigarette smoking make the diagnosis of α_1-antitrypsin (AAT) deficiency most likely. He probably has the homozygous ZZ genotype that causes a marked reduction of AAT levels to <15% normal. The radiograph is consistent with panacinar emphysema and alveolar destruction predominantly at the bases. The lung destruction is due to release of proteolytic enzymes from neutrophils and other inflammatory cells in response to environmental stimuli. These enzymes are normally neutralized by the antiproteases in the lung to prevent lung destruction in the presence of mild inflammatory stimuli. In AAT deficiency, the proteases are not neutralized, and induce panacinar emphysema under 'normal' circumstances. Cigarette smoking induces a neutrophilic response in the lung that accelerates the decline of lung function in AAT deficiency. Intravenous replacement of AAT in patients with reduced lung function may slow the decline in FEV_1.

Case 4: Restrictive ventilatory defect

1 Both patients have restrictive ventilatory defects based on the reduced TLC. FEV_1 and FVC are reduced proportionally, so the FEV_1/FVC is normal; therefore there is no obstructive ventilatory defect. Patient A has reduced $D_L CO$, signifying a gas transfer defect.

2 Restrictive ventilatory defects may be due to stiff lungs, stiff chest wall or weak respiratory muscles. Diseases causing stiff lungs will reduce all lung volumes/capacities simultaneously, including TLC, FRC and RV. Most parenchymal lung diseases will also cause a reduced $D_L CO$, whereas chest wall disease and respiratory muscle disease will not. An increased RV is also not compatible with stiff lungs. Thus, Patient A seems to have a problem with stiff lungs. The relatively normal FRC and $D_L CO$ in Patient B suggest that the lungs and chest wall are normal. Either a stiff chest wall or weak muscles may cause an increased RV. Patient B's lung function and difficulty in rising out of a chair and raising his arms suggest a muscle disease. Diseases causing weak respiratory muscles will reduce TLC, because the patient cannot inspire deeply.

3 The FRC is determined by the balance between the inward pull of the lung elastic recoil pressure and the outward pull of the chest wall. Therefore, FRC will be reduced if either the net lung recoil pressure increases (due to stiff, low compliance lungs), or if the net outward pull of the chest wall decreases (e.g. when scarring of the chest wall produces an added inward recoiling force). Since FRC is determined by the balance between two opposing static forces, respiratory muscle weakness should not influence FRC. However, in clinical practice, patients with respiratory muscle weakness often have a slightly reduced FRC. The mechanism for this finding is probably related to the lack of deep breaths or sighs causing microatelectasis that will increase lung recoil and decrease compliance.

RV is the amount of gas remaining in the lung at the end of maximal expiration. In adults, RV is determined by airway collapse at low lung volumes. However, this presupposes adequate expiratory muscle strength to actively lower lung volume below FRC (which can be reached from TLC passively). Patient A has normal muscle strength and airways that resist collapse due to the parenchymal lung disease, resulting in a reduced RV. Patient B has weak expiratory muscles, resulting in an elevated RV.

4 The differential diagnosis is long, and includes the disorders discussed in Chapter 29. Briefly, these would include occupational/environmental disorders, connective tissue/autoimmune diseases, drug/treatment-induced diseases, primary lung disorders or idiopathic disorders. Idiopathic pulmonary fibrosis or cryptogenic fibrosing alveolitis is likely in a 60-year-old with lung crackles, clubbing, no significant past history, no signs or symptoms of extrapulmonary disease and the lung function shown for Patient A.

5 Respiratory muscle weakness may be due to a variety of neuromuscular diseases that can involve the spinal cord, motor nerves, neuromuscular junction or skeletal muscles:

- Spinal cord: tumour, syringomyelia, polio, amyotrophic lateral sclerosis, tetanus.
- Motor nerves: brachial/phrenic nerve neuritis, trauma.
- Neuromuscular junction: myasthenia gravis, botulism, organophosphate poisoning.
- Skeletal muscle: muscular dystrophy, myositis, mitochondrial disease, myopathy (nutritional, drug, metabolic, inherited).

6 Hypoxaemia in interstitial lung diseases is usually due to ventilation–perfusion mismatching. Patient A likely has hypocapnia, because patients with interstitial lung disease tend to hyperventilate in response to stiff lungs and hypoxia. This will lower arterial carbon dioxide tension. In contrast, Patient B likely has hypoxaemia due to alveolar hypoventilation, and is therefore hypercapnic. Patient B is also more likely to develop acute respiratory failure with the limited ventilatory reserve due to the muscle weakness.

Case 5: Haemoptysis

1 The table below illustrates that most cases of haemoptysis are due to infection (~80%)—including tuberculosis, pneumonia, lung abscess and bronchiectasis. Only a minority are due to malignancy (~20%). Pulmonary embolism and trauma are other potentially important causes. The bronchial (rather than the pulmonary) circulation is the usual source of bleeding.

2 Approximately 35–40% of cases of haemoptysis are classified as trivial (flecks of blood in sputum), 45–50% as moderate (<500 mL or 0.5–2 cups daily) and only 10–20% as massive (>500 mL or more than 2 cups of blood daily). Mortality is directly related to the rate and volume of blood loss and the underlying pathology. In patients expectorating >500 mL of blood within a 4-h period, the mortality is ~70%, compared with 5% in patients expectorating the same quantity over 16–48 h. Death results from asphyxia, caused by flooding of the alveoli and only rarely from circulatory collapse.

3 A good history is essential, and may indicate the cause of haemoptysis. The characteristic clinical picture of diseases such as tuberculosis, bronchiectasis and bronchogenic carcinoma may direct subsequent investigation and management. Chest examination may reveal localized crepitations or consolidation but widespread soiling of the

Infective (~80%)	Malignant (~20%)	Other
Tuberculosis	Lung cancer	Pulmonary infarction
Pneumonia	Metastatic cancer	Adenoma
Lung abscess	Lymphoma	Traumatic
Bronchiectasis		Alveolar haemorrhage
Aspergillus		Vasculitis

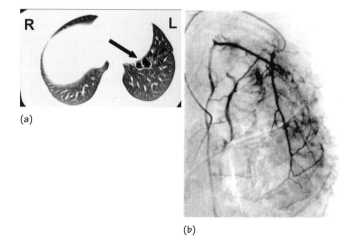

(a)

(b)

Fig. 45 (a) CT scan, (b) bronchial arteriography.

tracheobronchial tree with blood (due to coughing) often results in diffuse clinical signs. Examination of expectorated blood may provide clues. Food particles suggest the possibility of haematemesis, but blood in the nasogastric aspirate does not differentiate between haematemesis and haemoptysis, as coughed-up blood is often swallowed. Purulent material in the sputum may indicate bronchiectasis or a lung abscess. Associated haematuria raises the possibility of an alveolar haemorrhage syndrome. In this case, the age of the patient, the long history of minor haemoptysis and the symptoms of purulent sputum and night-time fever suggest a diagnosis of **bronchiectasis**, although other potential causes include recurrent pulmonary emboli, vasculitis and a benign adenoma.

4 Routine blood tests (white cell count raised in infection), including erythrocyte sedimentation rate (ESR) (raised in vasculitis) and C-reactive protein (raised in infection). Specialist blood tests (D-dimers for pulmonary emboli, *Aspergillus* precipitans, vasculitis screen) may be required. Sputum microbiology may isolate infective organisms (pneumonia, abscess, *Aspergillus*) or acid-fast bacilli (tuberculosis). A screening Heaf test may detect tuberculosis. Chest radiography should be obtained in all patients. It may provide important diagnostic information including evidence of a mass, cavity or abscess. CT scans with contrast may detect the site of bleeding, tumours, vascular malformations and other structural abnormalities. In this case, the CT scan demonstrated a grossly dilated bronchus (>10 mm) consistent with bronchiectasis in the anteromedial segment of the left lower lobe (Fig. 45a). Bronchoscopy is often required to detect endobronchial lesions and inhaled objects (e.g. tooth). Combinations of bronchoscopy and CT scanning have the highest diagnostic yield. Bronchial arteriography may be required to detect the site of bleeding (Fig. 45b).

5 Bronchiectasis is described in Chapter 32.

6 The key aspects of management of massive haemoptysis are to maintain a patent airway and oxygenation (oxygen therapy). Asphyxia (not bleeding) is the greatest immediate risk to the patient. Promote drainage of blood and prevent alveolar 'soiling' by positioning the patient slightly head down in the lateral decubitus position, with the 'presumed' bleeding side down. Determine the cause, site and severity of the bleeding (as above): haematemesis and upper airways bleeding (e.g. nose) may be confused with haemoptysis. Treatment of the underlying cause is essential if the haemoptysis is to be controlled (antibiotics for pneumonia or a lung abscess). Avoid excessive chest manipulation, including physiotherapy, as this may increase or restart bleeding. Cough suppression with codeine 30–60 mg every 6 h may be helpful. Institute appropriate antibiotics and bronchodilators.

Immediate control of haemoptysis is achieved at bronchoscopy by directing boluses of iced saline with epinephrine (10 mL; 1 : 10 000 dilution) at the bleeding site.

Bronchial angiography and embolization are the established therapeutic techniques for the initial control of haemoptysis. This procedure is initially successful in 70–100% of cases. The best results are described in patients with dilated bronchial arteries (e.g. bronchiectasis). Rebleeding often occurs (~40%), and infarction of the anterior spinal artery with paraplegia is reported (~5%). Most studies agree that surgical therapy is associated with the best long-term outcomes for isolated lesions. Primary medical management may be mandatory because bleeding cannot be localized (widespread *Aspergillus* infection) or is not amenable to surgical resection of a pulmonary segment. In other patients, surgery will be contraindicated because of end-stage lung disease ($FEV_1 < 40\%$ predicted), poor cardiac reserve, unresectable cancer or severe bleeding diathesis.

Final diagnosis: bronchiectasis of the anteromedial segment of the left lower lobe.

Index

at a Glance

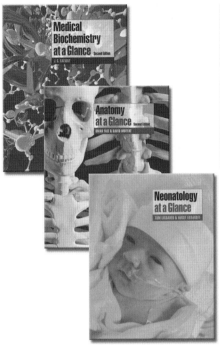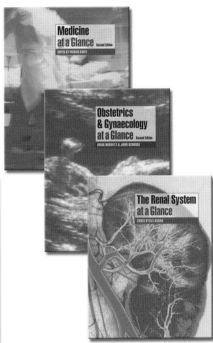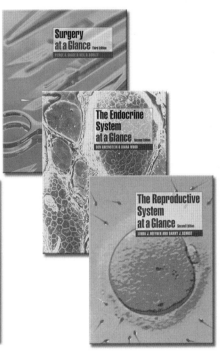

- The most simple and concise approach to all your subjects
  - Each bite-sized chapter covered in a double-page spread with key facts and fundamentals and a summary diagram
    - Perfect for exam preparation and use on clinical rotations

Titles in the at a Glance series

- Anatomy at a Glance
- The Cardiovascular System at a Glance
- Critical Care Medicine at a Glance
- The Endocrine System at a Glance
- The Gastrointestinal System at a Glance
- Haematology at a Glance
- History and Examination at a Glance
- Immunology at a Glance
- Medical Biochemistry at a Glance
- Medical Genetics at a Glance
- Medical Microbiology and Infection at a Glance
- Medical Pharmacology at a Glance
- Medical Statistics at a Glance

- Medicine at a Glance
- Metabolism at a Glance
- Neonatology at a Glance
- Neuroscience at a Glance
- Obstetrics and Gynaecology at a Glance
- Ophthalmology at a Glance
- Paediatrics at a Glance
- Physiology at a Glance
- Psychiatry at a Glance
- The Renal System at a Glance
- The Reproductive System at a Glance
- The Respiratory System at a Glance
- Surgery at a Glance

www.blackwellmedstudent.com

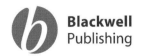

Blackwell Publishing

LECTURE NOTES

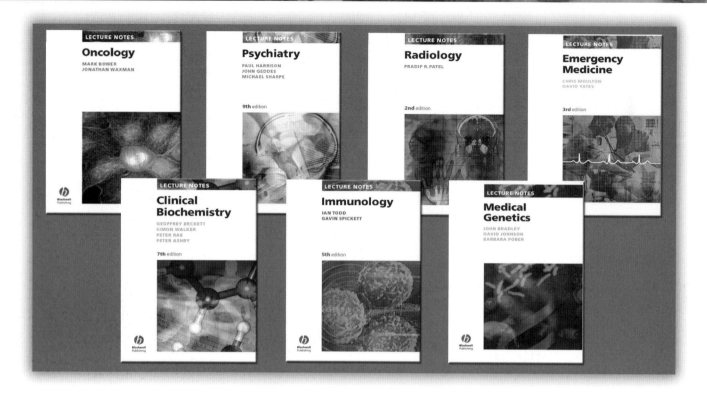

- Concise learning guides for all your subjects
- Focused on what you need to know
- Tried and Trusted

Titles in the LECTURE NOTES series

- Cardiology
- Clinical Anaesthesia
- Clinical Biochemistry
- Clinical Medicine
- Clinical Pharmacology and Therapeutics
- Clinical Skills
- Dermatology
- Diseases of the Ear, Nose and Throat
- Emergency Medicine

- Epidemiology and Public Health Medicine
- General Surgery
- Geriatric Medicine
- Haematology
- Human Physiology
- Immunology
- Infectious Diseases
- Medical Law and Ethics
- Medical Microbiology
- Molecular Medicine

- Neurology
- Obstetrics and Gynaecology
- Oncology
- Opthalmology
- Orthopaedics and Fractures
- Paediatrics
- Psychiatry
- Radiology
- Respiratory Medicine
- Tropical Medicine
- Urology

www.blackwellmedstudent.com

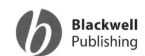

Blackwell Publishing

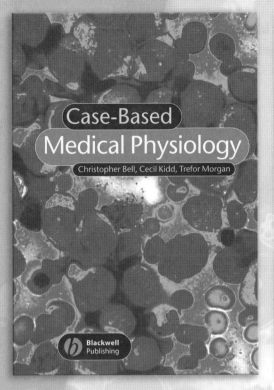
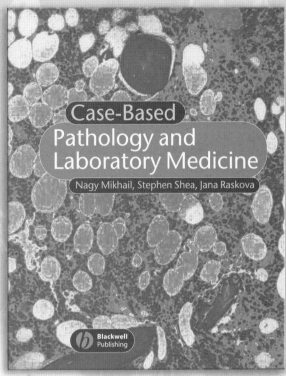
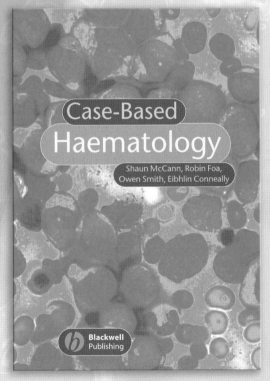
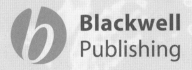

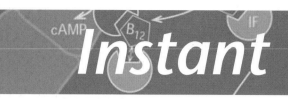

Instant

- **Each topic concisely presented in a double-page spread**

- **Indispensable core basic science 'dip in' revision aids**

- **Concentrates on key topics for finals and college examinations**

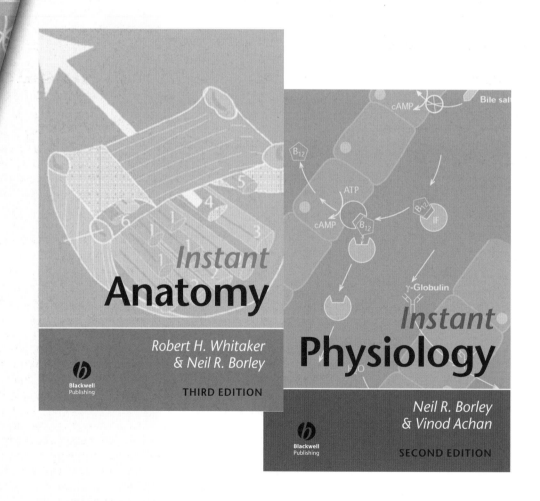

Instant
Anatomy

*Robert H. Whitaker
& Neil R. Borley*

Blackwell
Publishing

THIRD EDITION

Instant
Physiology

*Neil R. Borley
& Vinod Achan*

Blackwell
Publishing

SECOND EDITION

Titles in series: Anatomy • Clinical Pharmacology • Pathology • Physiology